D0567357

# Alzheimer's Disease

## Recent Titles in the Biographies of Disease Series

Influenza
*Roni K. Devlin*

ADHD
*Paul Graves Hammerness*

Food Allergies
*Alice C. Richer*

Anorexia
*Stacy Beller Stryer*

Obesity
*Kathleen Y. Wolin, Sc.D. and Jennifer M. Petrelli*

Sports Injuries
*Jennifer A. Baima*

Polio
*Daniel J. Wilson*

Cancer
*Susan Elaine Pories, Marsha A. Moses, and Margaret M. Lotz*

Fibromyalgia
*Kim D. Jones and Janice H. Hoffman*

Alcoholism
*Maria Gifford*

Anxiety
*Cheryl Winning Ghinassi*

Thyroid Disease
*Sareh Parangi and Roy Phitayakorn*

# Alzheimer's Disease

Linda C. Lu and Juergen H. Bludau

Biographies of Disease
*Julie K. Silver, M.D., Series Editor*

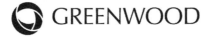 GREENWOOD

AN IMPRINT OF ABC-CLIO, LLC
Santa Barbara, California • Denver, Colorado • Oxford, England

**Library of Congress Cataloging-in-Publication Data**

Lu, Linda C.
    Alzheimer's disease / Linda C. Lu and Juergen H. Bludau.
      p. ; cm. — (Biographies of disease)
    Includes bibliographical references and index.
    ISBN 978-0-313-38110-2 (alk. paper) — ISBN 978-0-313-38111-9 (ebook)
1. Alzheimer's disease.   I. Bludau, Juergen.   II. Title.   III. Series: Biographies of disease. 1940-445X
    [DNLM:   1. Alzheimer Disease—etiology.   2. Alzheimer Disease—diagnosis.
3. Alzheimer Disease—therapy. WT 155]
    RC523.L8   2011
    616.8'31—dc22      2010041534

ISBN: 978-0-313-38110-2
EISBN: 978-0-313-38111-9

15  14  13  12  11    1  2  3  4  5

This book is also available on the World Wide Web as an eBook.
Visit www.abc-clio.com for details.

Greenwood
An Imprint of ABC-CLIO, LLC

ABC-CLIO, LLC
130 Cremona Drive, P.O. Box 1911
Santa Barbara, California 93116-1911

This book is printed on acid-free paper ∞

Manufactured in the United States of America

# Contents

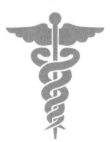

Series Foreword                                                                    vii

Preface                                                                             ix

Introduction                                                                        xi

Chapter 1. What Is Alzheimer's Disease?                                             1

Chapter 2. What Causes Alzheimer's Disease?                                         15

Chapter 3. What Are the Signs of Alzheimer's Disease?                              27

Chapter 4. How Is Alzheimer's Disease Diagnosed?                                   39

Chapter 5. How Is Alzheimer's Disease Treated?                                     59

Chapter 6. The Course and Complications of Alzheimer's Disease                     79

Chapter 7. How Does Alzheimer's Disease Affect
           the Family and Caregivers?                                              89

Chapter 8. Scientific and Clinical Research in Alzheimer's Disease                 103

Appendix A. Narratives                                    111

Appendix B. Timeline                                      123

Appendix C. 10 Useful Web Sites                           127

*Glossary*                                                131

*Bibliography*                                            133

*Index*                                                   139

# Series Foreword

E very disease has a story to tell: about how it started long ago and began to disable or even take the lives of its innocent victims, about the way it hurts us, and about how we are trying to stop it. In this Biographies of Disease series, the authors tell the stories of the diseases that we have come to know and dread.

The stories of these diseases have all of the components that make for great literature. There is incredible drama played out in real-life scenes from the past, present, and future. You'll read about how men and women of science stumbled trying to save the lives of those they aimed to protect. Turn the pages and you'll also learn about the amazing success of those who fought for health and won, often saving thousands of lives in the process.

If you don't want to be a health professional or research scientist now, when you finish this book you may think differently. The men and women in this book are heroes who often risked their own lives to save or improve ours. This is the biography of a disease, but it is also the story of real people who made incredible sacrifices to stop it in its tracks.

Julie K. Silver, M.D.
Assistant Professor, Harvard Medical School
Department of Physical Medicine and Rehabilitation

# Preface

This book provides the reader with a comprehensive, clinically sound, yet easy to understand overview of Alzheimer's disease. The more we understand about this disease, the more complicated it appears to become. What we do know, and increasingly recognize, is that Alzheimer's disease is becoming a major concern to the health care system of any society. For this reason it is even more important to know as much about this disease as possible. Only then will we be better at recognizing and ultimately supporting people who suffer from it.

To this extent the book starts with a general introduction to Alzheimer's disease and how it disrupts brain function. This is followed by a summary of the currently known risk factors for the disease and the classical symptoms and disease course people usually present with. The diagnosis and treatment options are discussed in detail and particular emphasis is placed on the effect the disease has on the family and caregivers. The book ends with a look at the current research into the disease and some promising future treatment options.

Using case studies as examples along the way makes the book come alive and the disease as real to the reader as it is to the patients and their caregivers.

# Introduction

From the Staedtische Anstalt fuer Irre und Epileptische in Frankfurt, Germany (Asylum for Lunatics and Epileptics) to the White House in Washington D.C., Alzheimer's disease has made its debut to become a global threat to an ever-increasing older population. As we know today, almost exactly 100 years apart, a German housewife named Auguste Deter in 1906 and the 40th president of the United States of America, Ronald Reagan, in 1994, were both diagnosed with the same disease that affected their brains. If it had not been for the curious mind of Dr. Alois Alzheimer, a German psychiatrist and neuropathologist, Auguste Deter would have never been diagnosed with a disease that ultimately carried his name. Upon her death Dr. Alzheimer and his colleague Emil Kraepelin dissected Auguste's brain and noticed several striking features which had not been described before. Among them were a stunning shrinkage of the entire brain and both dense deposits surrounding the nerve cells (amyloid plaques) and intracellular damage (neurofibrillary tangles). Despite the publication of his findings, the disease as we know it seemed to have been forgotten after Alzheimer's death in 1915 only to reemerge in the 1970s as the medical community recognized that this disease is not just simply a normal part of aging.

Since then the disease has affected millions of people around the world. Among them actress Rita Hayworth, actor Charles Bronson, former British prime minister Harold Wilson, and French fashion designer Louis Feraud, to name just a few well-known people. Great progress has been made in identifying risk factors, and accurately diagnosing the disease. However, despite millions of dollars spent yearly on research and thousands of researchers and clinicians around the world working on an effective treatment, a cure has so far been elusive. As a result, the dreaded "A" word, as it is often called by patients and caregivers alike, keeps haunting mankind.

# 1

# What Is Alzheimer's Disease?

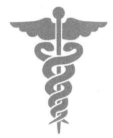

**November 1901 Frankfurt, Germany**

*She sits on the bed with a helpless expression. What is your name?*
  *Auguste.*
  *Last name?*
  *Auguste.*
  *What is your husband's name?*
  *Auguste, I think.*
  *Your husband?*
  *Ah, my husband.*
  *She looks as if she didn't understand the question. Are you married?*
  *To Auguste.*
  *Mrs. D?*
  *Yes, yes, Auguste D.*
  *How long have you been here? She seems to be trying to remember.*
  *Three weeks.*
  *What is this? I show her a pencil.*
  *A pen.*

T his is an excerpt taken from Dr. Alois Alzheimer's notes on conversations between him and Auguste D. (Maurer 1997). Auguste D. was a 51-year old German housewife who became a patient of Dr. Alzheimer's in 1901. She was admitted to a Frankfurt hospital for increasing confusion and memory loss. She was also paranoid that her husband was having an affair. Furthermore, she was hearing voices. Auguste D. eventually became bedridden and lost control of her bladder function, which is known as becoming incontinent. She died five years later, in 1906, of overwhelming infections from bedsores and pneumonia. After her death, Dr. Alzheimer received permission from her family to autopsy her brain. Examining her brain under a microscope, he described findings of unusual clumps (now known as amyloid plaques) and fiber tangles that would become synonymous with her disease. Auguste D.'s illness was eventually named after her physician, Dr. Alzheimer.

Alzheimer's disease is a progressive and fatal disease of the brain. It is a degenerative disease of the brain that leads to a condition called dementia. Dementia is a general term used to describe the loss of memory and mental abilities severe enough to affect daily life. Alzheimer's disease is the most common type of dementia, comprising 60 to 80 percent of all dementias. Because of this, the word "dementia" is sometimes used interchangeably with Alzheimer's disease. However, there are other types of dementia as well, such as vascular, Lewy body, or frontotemporal, just to name a few. We will not go into detail about the other types of dementia, but just keep in mind that dementia refers to a group of brain disorders, not only to Alzheimer's disease.

In order to function independently in our society, one must be able to perform certain basic activities, such as eating and grooming. When someone has dementia, the brain loses its ability to perform these basic skills. Let's take getting to work, for example. It is a simple act that millions of people perform daily without even thinking about the complexity of it. Average Joe would need to wake up in the morning, use the toilet, brush his teeth, pick out appropriate clothing, and put them on. Then, he would need to prepare and eat breakfast. And drive to work. All these tasks sound simple enough, and we frequently take the ability to carry them out for granted.

Now, what if Average Joe starts to have problems with his memory and thinking abilities? Imagine how these simple tasks can suddenly become difficult. How do you brush your teeth if you cannot remember how to use a toothbrush? What happens if you put on a T-shirt because you forget it is winter and snowing outside? How do you use a fork and knife if you cannot remember what they are? What happens if you scramble some eggs for breakfast and forget to turn off the stove? How do you drive to work if you do not remember the directions? These are examples of common problems encountered by people with dementia. It is losing cognitive and memory abilities to the point where it affects a person's ability to function independently in daily activities. As you can probably imagine, it is very scary to lose one's memories, especially if one is aware of this change. It is often quite difficult to cope, especially in someone who has been very independent.

When someone says "I'm getting Alzheimer's" jokingly, he usually means "I'm becoming forgetful." However, Alzheimer's disease is about more than just losing memory. It is a disease that damages all parts of the brain. It begins by impairing the memory center in the brain, and then progresses to the areas of the brain that control speech, vision, thinking, and reasoning. Over time, all brain functions are affected. Let's go back to Dr. Alzheimer's patient, Auguste D. She had memory problems early on. She had difficulty with remembering recent events, or even things said to her just minutes ago. "When objects are shown to her, she does not remember after a short time which objects have been shown." She developed language and word-finding difficulties. "When she was chewing meat and asked what she was doing, she answered *potatoes* and then *horseradish*." Her reasoning became altered. "If you buy 6 eggs, at 7 dimes each, how much is it? *Differently*."

As Alzheimer's disease progressed, the vision control center of Auguste D.'s brain became impaired. "She holds the book in such a way that one has the impression that she has a loss in the right visual field." She then started hearing voices as the disease spread to the part of the brain controlling hearing. "She suddenly says *Just now a child called, is he there?*" Auguste D. became paranoid and more and more confused. "[She] showed great fear and repeated *I will not be cut. I do not cut myself*." Then the areas of the brain coordinating her limb movements became damaged, and she stopped being able to walk. She became bedbound. She lost control of her bladder and bowels. At the end of the disease, death frequently is brought on by infections. Auguste D. developed overwhelming infection from bedsores and pneumonia, which are quite common in someone with end-stage Alzheimer's disease.

The course and duration of Alzheimer's disease varies from person to person. It depends on multiple factors, including the age of diagnosis and other medical problems that the person may have. On average, if the person is older, let's say after age 80, when the diagnosis is made, the disease course may only be three to four years. In someone younger, the disease from the time of diagnosis to death may be as long as 8 to 10 years or more. Frequently, family members notice small changes for many years before their loved one is brought to the doctor's office. The changes may be increased forgetfulness or small shifts in personality. Children or spouses will often attribute these subtle differences to "just old age." The patients themselves may or may not notice the changes.

Everyone responds to these cognitive changes differently. Some become very adept at hiding memory problems early on. For example, they will describe an object if they have trouble recalling its name. Or keep lists and calendars to help them remember dates and events. Others may not be aware of it, and vehemently deny any problems when family members express concern. It isn't usually until their cognitive impairments start affecting their ability to function in everyday life that patients themselves or family members become worried enough to seek medical help. Some examples of serious impairments include getting lost while driving home, forgetting the names of grandchildren, or no longer being able to balance their checkbooks.

## HOW MANY PEOPLE HAVE ALZHEIMER'S DISEASE?

More than 5 million Americans are currently living with Alzheimer's disease. That is more people than the entire population of New Zealand or Ireland. By 2050, it is expected that there will be 11 to 16 million people diagnosed with Alzheimer's disease in the United States. Almost 1 million people will be diagnosed annually. To put it another way, someone will develop this disease every 33 seconds (Alzheimer's Association 2009).

Alzheimer's disease is not exclusive to Americans. Worldwide, there were more than 26 million cases in 2006. The number of people affected is expected to be more than 100 million by 2050. That's nearly four times as many cases! But keep in mind that these numbers are only estimates based on diagnosis. Because some people do not seek medical help, the actual number of cases is likely higher. In an interesting side note, available data suggests that Alzheimer's disease may be more common in industrialized, western countries compared to countries in Asia and Africa (World Health Organization). Is this difference real? We do not know at this point. Several explanations for this discrepancy have been proposed. One is that the patients may be diagnosed with terms other than Alzheimer's disease, such as senility, and thus are not picked up by population studies. Another explanation could be a lack of knowledge about Alzheimer's disease when someone presents with it, so it goes undiagnosed. The lack of access to advanced medical care may shorten the length of survival of these people. Or it may be that people who live in Asia and Africa have protective factors that we still do not understand. Nonetheless, the prevalence of Alzheimer's disease throughout the world, on the whole, is on the rise.

One might wonder why the number of people with Alzheimer's disease is rising so rapidly, especially in the United States. This is because Alzheimer's disease occurs more frequently in older adults. And it is no secret that the U.S. population is growing older. Not only has life expectancy risen, but also the proportion of elderly people is growing rapidly. In the United States, people age 65 years and older currently make up about 13 percent of the population. They are projected to comprise 25 percent of the population by 2050. This means if you were to walk down the street, every fourth person you encounter will be older than age 65.

Because of new medications and advances in medical technology and medicines within the last century, people are living longer. Add to that a large increase in the number of births, and it is no surprise that our aging population is growing. This growth spurt is in part due to the aging baby boomers. The baby boom generation refers to the babies born in the decade or so after World War II, when there was a major surge in births. Before the baby boom period, it was difficult to raise children because of first, the Great Depression, and then World War II. After the war ended, there was a long period of peace and prosperity. Men returned from the war and rejoined the workforce. And many women left wartime jobs to bear and raise children. The first baby boomers turned 60 in 2006 (U.S. Census Bureau).

## COST OF ALZHEIMER'S DISEASE

Along with the increasing number of people with Alzheimer's disease is the associated cost of caring for them. It is very expensive. The most recent estimate puts the cost at more than $94 billion a year in Medicare costs for people with Alzheimer's disease who live at home. (Alzheimer's Association 2009). Medicare is government health insurance for people over the age of 65. Some younger people with certain disabilities or anyone with kidney failure can qualify as well. However, almost 90 percent of Medicare enrollees are seniors (Centers for Medicare and Medicaid Services). In addition to the medical expenditures involved in caring for Alzheimer's patients in the community, there is also the cost of nursing home care. The most recent estimate was more than $21 billion a year in nursing home costs for Alzheimer's patients (Alzheimer's Association 2009).

The majority of care provided to people with Alzheimer's disease is in the community. Who are the caregivers? Usually, it's a family member, either a spouse or child. Sometimes it can be a close relative. At times, the patient may live alone, with the assistance of home services. However, this is usually only if he or she has early disease. At last estimate, there are almost 10 million unpaid caregivers in the United States (Alzheimer's Association 2009). That's as many people as the entire population of the state of Michigan or the country of Portugal. These are the husbands, wives, daughters, sons, and grandchildren who provide care at home to their loved ones with Alzheimer's disease. They may live with the person or travel to take care of them. Ten percent of caregivers live more than two hours away. These unpaid caregivers provide countless hours of care, day and night, that we can't a put a price tag on. In 2008, these unpaid caregivers provided a total of 8.5 *billion* hours of care. If these unpaid caregivers were actually to be compensated for their time, at an average rate of $11 per hour, it would amount to almost $94 billion. This is even more than the cost of actual medical care provided to Alzheimer's patients.

Not only is treating Alzheimer's disease a significant cost to the health care system, it also has a profound impact on the lives of their caregivers. Keep in mind that a lot of these caregivers also work full-time jobs. One study puts the cost at $36.5 billion in indirect costs—such as lost productivity and the cost of paying another worker to perform their job if they are absent—to business for employees who are caregivers of people with Alzheimer's disease and other forms of dementia (Alzheimer's Association and National Alliance for Caregiving). Not only is treating Alzheimer's disease a significant cost to the health care system, it also has a profound impact on the lives of their caregivers.

## THE BRAIN

Before we learn about the brain changes in Alzheimer's disease, let's first talk about the basic workings of the brain. The human brain is an intricate organ that carries out many crucial tasks. It is the control center that directs all major functions in the body. By doing so, it allows us to live, breathe, and carry out the functions needed to lead our daily lives. The amount of work done by this organ, the size of a cantaloupe, is quite amazing. Besides controlling breathing, it allows us to think, see, hear, and move. It allows us to make and store memories. It also permits us to feel emotions.

How is the brain able to carry out all these functions? It does so through a complicated system of chemical and electrical processes. These chemical and electrical reactions are carried out by nerve cells, or neurons. There are approximately 100 billion neurons in the human brain. Each neuron is like a miniature computer. It receives, processes, generates, and transmits information. In order for it to function properly, its battery needs to be charged, and faulty or unnecessary information is thrown into the delete bin. In Alzheimer's disease, various parts of the neuron's hardware start breaking down. Scientists are working very hard to figure out exactly where the problem starts. As you can imagine, malfunctioning of one part, whether it be a jam in information processing or lack of energy supply, can bring the neuron's machinery to a screeching halt. The neuron stops carrying out its job and eventually dies.

These nerve cells are able to carry out their functions with the assistance and nourishment from support cells. The most abundant type of support cell is called the glial cell. Glial cells are motherly cells. They act as insulation and keep the neurons in place, provide them with nutrients, and clean up after them by disposing of cellular debris, and rid the brain of damaged cells. Another major component of the brain are the blood vessels. Billions of tiny blood vessels, also known as capillaries, make up a complex network of blood vessels in the brain. The brain consumes 20 percent of the body's blood supply even though it only makes up about 2 percent of the body's weight (National Institute on Aging). Later on, we will discuss how damages to this blood supply affect brain function.

Each neuron is made up of a cell body, an axon, and multiple dendrites. The axon is like an arm branching out from the cell body and transmits messages to neighboring neurons. It allows neurons to communicate with each other. Dendrites are like tentacles. They also extend from the cell body and receive messages from the axons of other neurons. Thus, axons send messages and dendrites receive messages.

Signals are transmitted from neuron to neuron via chemical or electrical mediators. When an axon sends a message to a neighboring neuron, it is in the form of chemical messengers that are released at the tip of the axon. There is a tiny gap between the axon tip and the dendrite that it is communicating with. This gap is called a synapse. Chemical messengers, or neurotransmitters (neuro = brain, transmitters = messengers) are released from the axon into the synapse. The neurotransmitters float across the synapse and dock at receptors on the receiving dendrite. Like a lock and key, there is a specific receptor for each type of neurotransmitter. When the neurotransmitter slides into its proper receptor, an electric impulse is initiated and propelled from the cell body to its axon, and the message is propagated to the next neuron. This is how neurons communicate with each other.

Not all neurons are the same. Each type of neuron has a particular job. For example, some neurons are responsible for thinking and making memory. Other neurons are specialized in receiving and processing information from the eyes, nose, or ears. Another group of neurons have the important task of signaling the muscles to move, such as talking or walking. Similar types of neurons are usually grouped together into the same location in the brain. In this way, particular brain functions can be localized to certain areas of the brain.

The brain consists of three major components, the cerebrum, cerebellum, and brain stem. The cerebrum controls movement and is involved in thinking, memories, and feelings. The cerebellum sits beneath the cerebrum at the back of the brain and is involved in balance and coordination. The brain stem connects the brain to the spinal cord and has important functions in regulating the body.

The cerebrum (Latin for brain) consists of two hemispheres, the right and left cerebral hemispheres. The billions of neurons in both hemispheres are connected by a large bundle of nerve fibers called the corpus callosum. The corpus callosum, "hard body" in Latin, is the largest bundle of nerve fibers in the entire human body. It allows the left and right cerebral hemispheres to communicate with each other. The outer layer of the cerebral hemispheres is called the cerebral cortex. Cortex means bark in Latin (as you have probably noticed, a lot of medical terminology is rooted in Latin), and like the bark of a tree, the cortex is the outer layer of the brain.

If we take a pen and draw imaginary lines through the cortex, we can divide each hemisphere into four lobes, each with special functions. The four lobes are frontal, parietal, temporal, and occipital. The lobe at the front of the brain is called the frontal lobe. Like an executive in a big corporation, it controls the "executive functions" of the brain. It makes the major decisions. Activities such as thinking, planning, problem-solving, and organizing occur in the frontal lobe. It also plays a role in executing movement. The *parietal lobe* is located behind the frontal lobe. It deals with sensation and perception. It integrates information from the sensory organs, and allows us to appreciate the different senses, such as smell or touch.

Next, let's discuss the *temporal lobe*. It sits under the frontal and parietal lobes. The temporal lobe is involved in the creation and storage of memories. It plays a role in coordinating the senses of sound, smell, and taste, as well. The last of the four lobes is the *occipital lobe*, situated at the back of the brain. Its main duty is vision. So there are four lobes on each side of the brain, each with special functions.

Buried underneath the cortex are structures that are also crucial to brain functioning. This network of structures is called the limbic system. The limbic system is composed of the amygdala, hippocampus, thalamus, and hypothalamus. Do not worry about trying to remember these odd-sounding names. The reason we are discussing them is because their important jobs are affected by Alzheimer's disease. In order to understand what happens when these structures malfunction, it's important to learn what their normal functions are first.

The *amygdala*, or almond in Latin, is an almond-shaped structure in the temporal lobe. Just remember one word associated with it—fear. Remember that funny feeling in your stomach the last time you watched a scary movie where someone was hiding in the dark about to pounce on the unsuspecting victim—or the butterflies in your stomach the last time you had to give a presentation in front of your class. The amygdala is responsible for those feelings. It both processes and stores strong emotions.

The *hippocampus*, or sea horse in Latin, sits behind the amygdala in the temporal lobe. It is a key structure in memory. It is involved in learning and re-

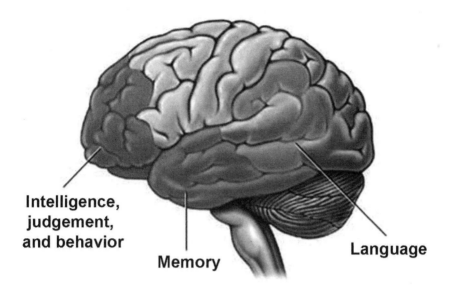

**Intelligence,
judgement,
and behavior**

**Memory**

**Language**

Different areas of the brain are responsible for certain functions. The temporal lobe is important in memory. (Courtesy of ABC-CLIO)

membering, especially short-term memory. Scientists believe it is the center for converting short-term memory into long-term memory, which is filed in other parts of the brain.

The significance of the hippocampus's role in memory was exemplified by the famous patient H.M., of Hartford, Connecticut. He suffered from intractable seizures, and in 1953, had parts of his brain surgically removed, including most of his hippocampus. After the surgery, he developed severe anterograde (forward direction) amnesia, meaning he lost the ability to commit new information to long-term memory. For example, you could have a coherent conversation with him. But if you left the room and came back an hour later, he would not remember you or the conversation. He also suffered from retrograde (backward direction) amnesia, and could not remember some events up to 11 years prior to his surgery. H.M.'s memory impairment after his surgery gave us better insight into certain areas of the brain that are involved in the complex workings of memory. As you have probably already deduced, the hippocampus becomes damaged in Alzheimer's disease. We will discuss this more later on.

Another structure within the limbic system is the *thalamus* (bridal couch in Latin), which sits on top of the brain stem. It is like the central processing center of the limbic system. It receives limbic and sensory information, processes them, and distributes the information to the cerebral cortex. Right beneath the thalamus is the *hypothalamus* (hypo=under). The main role of the hypothalamus is maintaining homeostasis, that is, the body's equilibrium. It monitors body activities such as body temperature, blood pressure, body weight, and fluid status, and keeps these systems close to a set point. It also controls the body's internal clock, as well as appetite.

## CHANGES TO THE BRAIN IN ALZHEIMER'S DISEASE

When Dr. Alzheimer examined Auguste D.'s brain under a microscope in 1906, he found two distinctly abnormal features—plaques and tangles. Scientists have since identified these two structures as hallmarks of Alzheimer's disease. Of course, the exact cause and process of Alzheimer's disease is still not well understood. Dedicated researchers are currently hard at work to decipher this disease, and hopefully, find a cure. We will discuss what findings have been discovered and are widely accepted thus far. Let's first review the changes at a cellular level. Then, we will talk about the overall brain changes as Alzheimer's disease progresses.

The abnormal plaques that develop in Alzheimer's disease are called amyloid plaques. The word "plaque" brings to mind an image of unsightly buildup on our teeth or in our blood vessels. The same can be said of amyloid plaques. Amyloid plaques are buildups of protein fragments called beta-amyloid, and these protein fragments are thought to be harmful to brain cells.

So where do these harmful beta-amyloids come from? Beta-amyloids originate from amyloid precursor proteins (APP). The APP is a large protein that is associated with the cell membrane, which is the outer layer of a cell, like an orange peel. It is sliced into smaller units by one of three enzymes. Depending on which enzyme does the cutting and where the cut is made, the APP is processed via different pathways. Beta-amyloids are created through one of these routes. The amyloid plaques are then deposited in the space between neurons and exert toxic effects on the neurons. Some people may develop plaques as a part of aging. However, in Alzheimer's disease, amyloid plaques tend to be more abundant in certain areas of the brain.

For many years, scientists believed that amyloid plaques were the potential culprits behind the neuronal damage seen in Alzheimer's disease. This thinking has since evolved, and it is still unclear whether amyloid plaques actually cause Alzheimer's disease, or whether they are a result of the disease process itself. There is some evidence to suggest that amyloid plaques may be an attempt by the brain to get the noxious beta-amyloid away from the nerve cells. We know that the beta-amyloid protein fragments cause damage to neurons. They tend to aggregate into larger units that react with neuron receptors and axons, thereby affecting the cell's ability to function. By clumping these beta-amyloid fragments, and adding other proteins and cellular materials, insoluble plaques form. In this way, the toxic beta-amyloids are quarantined. Whether the amyloid plaques cause or are produced by the dementia, they remain one of the distinctive characteristic brain findings in Alzheimer's disease.

Besides amyloid plaques, Dr. Alzheimer also noticed neurofibrillary tangles in Auguste D.'s brain. Neuro means brain, and fibrillary means fibers. So imagine looking through a microscope and finding a bunch of tangled, twisted fibers inside nerve cells. These fibers are made of proteins, the majority of which are *tau* (rhymes with how) proteins. A healthy neuron relies on several internal structures to maintain its functions. Microtubules (shaped like a stack of straws) play a key role in transporting nutrients and important cellular components. And tau proteins bind to these microtubules and stabilize them. In Alzheimer's disease, abnormal tau proteins break away from the microtubules and become twisted into tangles. Without the support of the tau proteins, the microtubules disassemble, and the internal network falters. The neuron becomes disabled, and is not longer able to function normally.

With the cumulative effects of amyloid plaques and neurofibrillary tangles over time, the neurons lose the ability to communicate with each other. As the disease progresses, and more and more neurons become injured and die, the affected parts of the brain start to shrink. This process is called brain atrophy and becomes more pronounced in the later stages of the disease.

As of right now, no one knows exactly when the disease process starts or what triggers its onset. Researchers believe the brain changes begin many years before symptoms are even suspected. They can start as long as 20 years or more prior to symptoms appearing.

Alzheimer's disease originates deep in the brain, in an area called the entorhinal cortex, next to the hippocampus. Amyloid plaques are deposited between neurons. The formation of neurofibrillary tangles inside neurons brings critical cell functions to a screeching halt. As the healthy neurons die off, the disease spreads to the neighboring hippocampus. Remember, the hippocampus is the main site for learning and remembering, especially forming short-term memories. One of the most frequent complaints about someone with early dementia is increased forgetfulness. Family members often complain about their repetitiveness because they have difficulty committing information to short-term memory and ask the same questions over and over again.

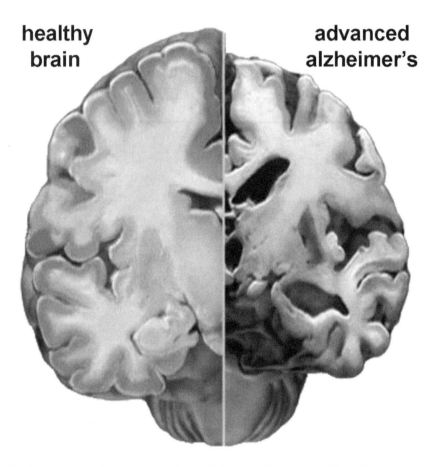

## healthy brain

## advanced alzheimer's

The brain changes that occur in Alzheimer's disease. (Courtesy of ABC-CLIO)

From the hippocampus, the disease spreads, and the plaques and tangles multiply throughout the brain. All the brain regions that we discussed earlier are affected, including the four lobes of the cerebral cortex, as well as the limbic system. The signs and symptoms of Alzheimer's disease become progressively more pronounced. And as the neurons die off, the brain begins to shrivel up like a prune. Ventricles, which are fluid-filled spaces within the brain, get bigger as the brain tissue shrinks. Finally, at the end stage of the disease, the brain looks like this (see photo). So as the brain dies, the rest of the body goes with it. This is the course of Alzheimer's disease.

Although this paints quite a bleak picture, there is a lot of exciting and innovative research being conducted in the field of Alzheimer's disease. Scientists are working hard to better understand Alzheimer's disease in all aspects. This includes studying the causes of Alzheimer's disease, developing better diagnostic tools, and creating potential new treatments.

# 2

# What Causes Alzheimer's Disease?

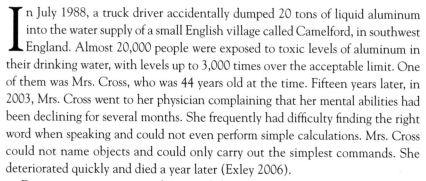

In July 1988, a truck driver accidentally dumped 20 tons of liquid aluminum into the water supply of a small English village called Camelford, in southwest England. Almost 20,000 people were exposed to toxic levels of aluminum in their drinking water, with levels up to 3,000 times over the acceptable limit. One of them was Mrs. Cross, who was 44 years old at the time. Fifteen years later, in 2003, Mrs. Cross went to her physician complaining that her mental abilities had been declining for several months. She frequently had difficulty finding the right word when speaking and could not even perform simple calculations. Mrs. Cross could not name objects and could only carry out the simplest commands. She deteriorated quickly and died a year later (Exley 2006).

During an autopsy, it was discovered that she had beta-amyloid proteins deposited in and around blood vessels throughout her brain. This distribution of beta-amyloid occurs in a rare type of Alzheimer's disease. She was also found to have more than 10 times the normal amount of aluminum in her brain.

So did the toxic aluminum exposure cause Mrs. Cross to develop Alzheimer's disease? The short answer is, we do not know. Forty years ago, aluminum exposure emerged as a potential cause of Alzheimer's disease. This led to great public concern as aluminum is used in numerous everyday items, such as foil, soda cans, and pots and pans. It can even be found in antiperspirants. However, many studies done since have been unable to show that aluminum plays any role in causing Alzheimer's disease. Currently, most experts do not think aluminum is a potential cause.

Numerous causes of Alzheimer's have been proposed over the years. There is controversy surrounding some of them, such as mercury or other so-called heavy metals or chemical exposure. This is a hot-button topic because if we can identify the cause, then theoretically, we can prevent the disease or use it as a target for treatment. But as of now, no single factor has been proven to directly cause Alzheimer's disease. The current thinking is that Alzheimer's disease is a complex process, involving many factors, that affect the brain over a long period of time. The factors include those that we inherit and those we acquire throughout life. Although an exact cause has not been identified, scientists have found several risk factors associated with Alzheimer's disease. A risk factor predisposes someone to developing the disease. This means that someone with a risk factor is more likely to get a disease than someone without it. Let's take a look at some of the known risk factors for Alzheimer's disease.

## FAMILIAL AND GENETIC FACTORS

Is Alzheimer's disease hereditary? This is one of the most frequently asked questions about Alzheimer's disease. For those people who have seen family members suffer from the disease, it can be quite a scary and worrisome prospect if the same fate awaits them. So if your grandmother or mother has it, does this mean you will get it? The answer is no, and yes. It is not hereditary in the sense that it is passed down directly from generation to generation. However, the risk of developing Alzheimer's disease increases if there is a "positive" family history. If an immediate family member has the disease, such as a parent or sibling, then the risk of developing it is two to three times greater than in someone without a family history.

The role that genetics plays in Alzheimer's disease is quite complex, and still not completely understood. What we do know is that having a first-degree relative—a parent or sibling—with the disease puts one at increased risk. Researchers have also learned from studying twins that the rate of both twins developing Alzheimer's disease is higher in identical twins than it is in fraternal twins. Now, recall that identical twins share the exact same copies of genes. So if there was a transmissible Alzheimer's gene, then we would expect that if one twin developed the disease, the other twin would also develop it 100 percent of the time, which we do not find. Not every twin gets the disease if his identical twin develops it. This suggests that in addition to genetics, other factors also play a role.

Several genetic mutations have been identified as being associated with Alzheimer's disease. A mutation is a change in the DNA. When a mutation occurs, it alters the gene's ability to carry out its regular function, and in some cases, can lead to detrimental effects, such as a birth defect or developing cancers.

Most cases of Alzheimer's disease are considered late-onset, meaning people typically get it in old age. However, in rare instances, it appears in younger people in their fifties or earlier. This is called early-onset familial Alzheimer's disease, which occurs in less than 10 percent of cases (Tanzi 1999). As the name suggests, people who get this form of Alzheimer's disease at an earlier age tend to have a strong family history of the disease. Up until now, researchers have identified three genetic mutations that are associated with early-onset Alzheimer's disease. The genetic mutations are in amyloid precursor protein, presenilin 1, and presenilin 2. Do not worry about remembering the names. The amyloid precursor protein should sound familiar from chapter 1. It is the protein from which beta-amyloids originate and from which amyloid plaques ultimately form.

In late-onset Alzheimer's disease, to date, only one gene has been discovered that poses significant risk: apolipoprotein E, or ApoE (pronounced ā -pō-ē). There are several variants of this genetic mutation, and the increased risk ranges anywhere from threefold to eightfold. This means that for someone carrying this genetic mutation, the risk of developing Alzheimer's disease can be as much as eight times higher than someone without this gene. ApoE is believed to account for almost half of all cases of late-onset Alzheimer's disease (Saunders 1993).

There is another group of people who are genetically susceptible to Alzheimer's disease—people with Down syndrome. Every human is born with two copies of each chromosome, 23 pairs in total. Down syndrome occurs when a person has three copies of chromosome 21, also known as trisomy (tri = three) 21. This extra copy of the 21st chromosome leads to developmental delays in physiologic growth and mental abilities. Almost all individuals with Down syndrome will develop Alzheimer's disease. Beta-amyloid plaques begin to form in the brain during childhood, as early as 8 years old in some cases (Leverenz 1998). The plaque buildup speeds up as the person gets older, and by age 40, virtually all adults with Down syndrome will have accumulated enough brain tissue damage to warrant a diagnosis of Alzheimer's disease (Lott 2005).

We have reviewed some familial and genetic risk factors for Alzheimer's disease. Having a family history is a strong risk factor. So are certain genetic mutations and having an extra copy of chromosome 21. But what is the most influential factor?

## AGE

Age is the biggest risk factor for Alzheimer's disease. Most people who develop Alzheimer's disease are older than age 65. The chance of getting Alzheimer's disease nearly doubles every five years after age 65. So by the time an individual reaches 85 years old, the risk of developing Alzheimer's disease is 16 times higher than it was at age 65 (Alzheimer's Association 2009). These statistics seem to suggest that the older one gets, the greater the chance of developing Alzheimer's disease. But remember, this is not a normal part of aging. Many people live into very old age with their mental abilities fully intact.

## HEAD INJURY

A head injury occurs when a hard blow to the head causes the brain to move about violently within the skull. The abrupt jarring of the brain can damage nerves, blood vessels, and brain tissue. The severity of the injury depends on the force and location of impact. Every year, close to one and a half million people in the United States suffer a head injury (Center for Disease Control). People who survive a traumatic brain injury may end up with permanent brain damage and neurological problems. Even mild damage to the brain can affect mental abilities.

Sugar Ray Robinson has been recognized by many as one of the best boxers who ever lived. During his illustrious career, he fought in more than 200 matches and won most of them. However, in the final years leading up to his death at age 67 in 1989, he was diagnosed with dementia. Dementia is a general term used to describe a group of syndromes characterized by the loss of mental abilities. Alzheimer's disease is the most common type of dementia. Sugar Ray Robinson is one example out of many professional boxers who have developed dementia pugilistica, the word for boxing in Latin.

Dementia pugilistica has been recognized for many years in boxers. Because they experience repeated blows to the head over a long period of time, boxers can develop chronic traumatic brain injuries. Dementia pugilistica is also known as punch drunk syndrome. With repeated jolts to the head, the resultant brain injuries lead to progressive impairment in memory and thinking abilities, not unlike dementia. These people will also develop an unsteady gait and problems with coordination. They may also have personality changes, with explosive or aggressive behavior. Thus, they tend to talk and behave as if they are "punch drunk." This is not a syndrome specific to just boxers. Professional athletes in high-contact sports such as football, wrestling, or hockey are also prone to developing dementia pugilistica.

For many years, dementia pugilistica was viewed as a degenerative brain disorder that was different from Alzheimer's disease. However, there is more data to suggest that traumatic brain injury can lead to changes in the brain similar to Alzheimer's disease. Thus, it can be a potential risk factor.

One of the earlier cases studied involved a young 22-year-old man who suffered a single episode of severe head trauma (Rudelli 1982). He made fairly good recovery, but in his thirties, he started to exhibit signs of dementia. After his death at age 38, an autopsy of his brain showed classic findings of Alzheimer's disease. Later studies of the brains of boxers who suffered from dementia pugilistica also showed beta-amyloid plaques, although they were not present in all the cases (Van Den Heuvel 2007). Researchers have also tried to look at how frequently people with traumatic brain injuries go on to develop dementia. Some studies have found a link, which is called a "positive association," but it was not seen in every case. Thus, there is an increasing amount of data to suggest that traumatic brain injury can be a risk factor for Alzheimer's disease, but the process is still not completely understood.

## VASCULAR RISK FACTORS

The human body relies on its circulatory system to function properly. The circulatory, or vascular, system is composed of blood vessels that carry blood to all the vital organs, such as heart, kidneys, liver, and brain. Just to give you an idea of how complex the vascular system is, think of it this way. If laid out in a straight line, the blood vessels of an adult human body would stretch out to almost 100,000 miles long! (The Franklin Institute). Put another way, it can be wrapped around the earth approximately four times! So, as you can see, our blood vessel system is quite intricate and complicated.

Blood vessels deliver oxygen-rich blood and nutrients to the critical organs and transport waste products away to be processed and removed from the body. The blood vessels in our body come in all sizes. Blood vessels that carry oxygen-rich blood from the heart to the rest of the body are called arteries. The heart pumps out blood into the largest artery in the body, called the aorta. As the blood is transported throughout the body, the arteries divide and split off into smaller and smaller sized vessels, until they reach the capillaries. The capillaries are the smallest blood vessels in the body; each capillary is so small the red blood cells can only go through it one by one, in single file. This is where the oxygen exchange occurs. Oxygen is released through the thin capillary walls, and waste products from the tissues are deposited into the blood to be carried away. There are capillary beds located throughout the entire body. The waste-carrying blood from the capillaries is carried away in blood vessels called veins.

So what does the vascular system have to do with dementia? Recall from the first chapter, it was mentioned that the brain consumes quite a big chunk of the body's blood supply. At least 20 percent of the body's blood supply goes to the brain even though it only makes up 2 percent of the body. So if there is any impediment to the blood getting to the brain, the brain's functions start faltering. Like a car running without oil, the engine will break down eventually.

Vascular disease is disease of the blood vessels. Vascular risk factors refer to certain medical conditions that can cause damage to the blood vessels. Injury to the blood vessels can affect the blood supply to the brain, and over time, lead to brain damage. These injuries to the brain can result in problems with memory and thinking abilities as seen in dementia. Many diseases can wound the blood vessels, but only a few medical conditions have been identified to be associated with an increased risk of Alzheimer's disease. However, keep in mind that these risk factors are just that, risk factors. Why they are potential risk factors is still not completely understood.

### Vascular Risk Factors: Hypertension

Hypertension means high blood pressure in medical lingo. Blood pressure is the force of the blood pushing against the arterial walls as the blood travels through the arteries. Imagine watering a lawn with a garden hose. If you squeeze and apply pressure on the hose, the water squirts out faster and harder. In hypertension, blood flows through the arteries in a similarly turbulent fashion. Normally, our blood pressure fluctuates throughout the day. It can be lower during sleep or rest. Blood pressure can become elevated when one feels anxious or after exercise, but it is expected to return to normal eventually. In hypertension, the blood pressure remains abnormally high, regardless of activities or other factors that can affect blood pressure. Over time, this high pressure leads to damage in the arteries and the organs that the arteries supply. The brain is one of the major organs affected.

Damage to the tiny blood vessels distributed throughout the brain means that delivery of oxygen and nutrients can be halted. Over time, starving brain tissues start to die off. In severe cases, a stroke—sudden loss of blood flow to the brain—occurs. Loss or damage to brain tissue in certain areas means losing particular functions. The changes can be subtle initially, but after years and decades, the person may start to exhibit personality or memory changes typically seen in dementia.

Hypertension has been linked to several types of dementia, in particular Alzheimer's and another type called vascular dementia. Several studies done to look at people with high blood pressure and whether they go on to develop dementia have found a positive association. But not all the studies have confirmed this association. The link between hypertension and Alzheimer's disease is not definitive. Not everyone with hypertension will develop Alzheimer's disease. But hypertension occurs more frequently in someone with Alzheimer's disease than in someone without it. Thus, high blood pressure is considered a risk factor, but it is not a definitive cause.

### Vascular Risk Factors: Hyperlipidemia

High cholesterol is a term frequently thrown around in the media, especially in television commercials and Internet ads for cholesterol medications. We probably all have relatives or know someone who is being treated for high cholesterol. So what is cholesterol? Cholesterol refers to fatty particles in our blood. It is a waxy, fatty substance that is found naturally in our blood and cells. Our body, in particular the liver, produces most of the cholesterol. Despite popular beliefs about diet, only a quarter of our cholesterol comes from the food we eat (American Heart Association).

Cholesterol plays an important part in normal body functions. For example, it is used to form cell membranes and some hormones. However, when the level of cholesterol becomes abnormally high, it starts causing problems with blood circulation. The medical terms for a high cholesterol level in the blood is hyperlipidemia (hyper = over, lipid = fat) or hypercholesterolemia. Undesirable fatty deposits can form plaques on the artery walls. This buildup causes narrowing of the blood vessels, which eventually reduces blood flow to vital organs. In severe cases, like backed-up plumbing, the blood flow can be severely restricted.

It is widely accepted that high cholesterol is associated with an increased risk of heart attack or stroke. But its role in Alzheimer's disease is unclear. Based on a few studies, high cholesterol may impose some risk for developing dementia (Solomon 2007). However, this is only a positive association, not definitive proof, and it has not been corroborated by some other studies. So, the research thus far has shown mixed results, and an association is unclear.

So what does all this mean? In a nutshell, high cholesterol may lead to an increased chance of developing Alzheimer's disease, but the association is not definitive. However, as with hypertension and other vascular risk factors, it may be beneficial to keep your cholesterol in check for overall dementia risk reduction.

### Vascular Risk Factors: Diabetes

Diabetes refers to abnormally high levels of glucose, or sugar, in the body. When food is digested and broken down, it triggers the pancreas to secrete insulin. The pancreas is an organ next to the stomach, and insulin is a hormone that is important in helping the body process glucose into energy for your body's cells. There are two types of diabetes. Type 1 diabetes typically occurs in youth. Type 2 diabetes occurs more frequently during middle age or beyond. We will focus on type 2 diabetes, as we will be discussing how it relates to Alzheimer's disease.

Type 2 diabetes occurs when the pancreas is unable to produce enough insulin to meet the body's demands. Frequently, the cells in the body also stop responding to insulin, called insulin resistance. Without enough insulin or adequate response to insulin, glucose builds up in the system. Over time, the body's inability to maintain normal levels of glucose and insulin can cause damage to various organs, including the brain.

It is well documented that someone with diabetes has a greatly increased risk for high blood pressure, high cholesterol, and, eventually, heart disease. The combination of diabetes, hypertension, hypercholesterolemia, and obesity are commonly referred to as the metabolic syndrome. It is no secret that the American population is getting heavier. Stereotypical images of overweight men and women are frequently depicted in the media. An obese person is likely to develop the metabolic syndrome, meaning he is at risk for high blood sugars, high blood pressure, and high cholesterol. In fact, the current thinking is that having diabetes is equivalent to having cardiovascular, or heart and vascular, disease. Diabetes carries a significant risk of developing problems with blood vessels. Recall the previous discussions regarding high blood pressure and high cholesterol, and how they may be risk factors for Alzheimer's disease. Well, if diabetes is highly associated with hypertension and hypercholesterolemia, then does it mean that it can also increase the chance of developing Alzheimer's dementia?

Several explanations to tie diabetes with dementia have been offered. Some animal studies have suggested that insulin may affect the metabolism of beta-amyloid and tau proteins (Biessels 2005). These proteins are thought to be involved in the formation of plaques and tangles found in the brains of Alzheimer's patients. Elevated levels of glucose in the brain may also have a damaging effect, but the mechanism is still not well understood. These are examples of proposed factors that may link diabetes and dementia, but the association is still not clear-cut.

Researchers have found that people with diabetes can develop impairments in their mental abilities over time (Gispen 2000). However, a deterioration in mental abilities does not necessarily mean that dementia is on the horizon. Several studies have demonstrated an affiliation between diabetes and Alzheimer's disease, and seem to suggest that someone with diabetes can be at risk for developing Alzheimer's disease later on (Arvanitakis 2004). They looked at people with and without diabetes, and determined how many of them were eventually diagnosed with Alzheimer's disease. There appears to be a higher percentage of people with diabetes than those without who go on to develop Alzheimer's disease. This would suggest that diabetes may put someone at increased risk for developing dementia later on in life. But, remember, this is only an association. Diabetes may be a potential risk factor for Alzheimer's disease, but more studies are needed to investigate this.

## LIFESTYLE AS A RISK FACTOR

We cannot change the genetic makeup we are born with. However, we can choose how to live our lives. Can personal decisions about how one chooses to live affect one's chances of getting Alzheimer's disease? This is a frequently asked question. If "lifestyle" choices have an effect on the risks of developing dementia, then theoretically, they can give those with a positive family history or genetic susceptibility a sense of hope.

What is meant by lifestyle? It is a very broad term that can encompass all aspects of daily living. There are three main components of lifestyle that we will discuss: mental activities, social activities, and physical activities. To live an enriched life, maintaining a social network and keeping fit physically and intellectually stimulated are important. Many studies have shown that maintaining these three lifestyle elements can improve overall health and prolong life. Furthermore, these three types of activities have been studied in relation to dementia risks, and there appears to be an association. An inverse association, that is. The risk of developing dementia is increased in those who are less active socially, mentally and physically (Fratiglioni 2004).

Mental activity refers to doing things that engage and challenge the mind, such as reading a book, playing an instrument, or doing crossword puzzles. Whenever mental activities are discussed, the role of education is frequently questioned. Does a higher education protect one from Alzheimer's disease, or on the other hand, does having a lower education predispose one to it? Some studies have looked into this, and the results suggest that those people with more formal education may be less likely to develop Alzheimer's disease (Stern 1994). A theory called "cognitive reserve" has been proposed to explain this effect. Think of a bank account. The more money you save, the more money is available for you to spend later on. With cognitive reserve, obtaining more education and mental stimulation during younger adulthood is like depositing into the "brain" account, so one has more mental abilities "reserved," or saved away. Thus, when the changes of Alzheimer's disease appear in the brain, a person with a higher cognitive reserve may be able to function longer before the dementia becomes apparent to the patient or family members (Ngandu 2007). However, once Alzheimer's disease is diagnosed, people with higher education tend to have a more rapid mental decline. This is likely in part because they have more disease changes in the brain by the time it is diagnosed, compared to someone with less education (Wilson 2004).

Physical activities are simply that, any activity that gets one off the couch and moving. It can be as simple as taking walks or gardening, or as strenuous as playing a sport. It can be any physical activity, as long as it increases the heart rate. The benefits of exercise are well-known and can help lower the risks of many medical conditions such as high blood pressure or diabetes, which are some of the vascular risk factors we discussed earlier.

In addition to mental and physical health, socializing is an important part of overall health. Social interaction with other people is an important part of being human. Recall the last time you met a new group of people, such as at a party or at school. Carrying on a conversation with someone unfamiliar is intellectually stimulating. It requires you to concentrate and take in new information, and think of something appropriate to say in response in order to continue the conversation. Interacting with other people also engages emotions, and brings comfort and affirmation that only human contact can offer.

Studies have shown that these various lifestyle factors can play a role in dementia risks (Fratiglioni 2004). Researchers have found that those people who are mostly sedentary are more likely to lose their cognitive or thinking abilities later in life. These people are more at risk for developing dementia later in life compared with people who get regular exercise or perform leisurely activities. The same is true for mental and social activities. People who stay active mentally throughout life by performing brain-stimulating tasks such as reading or pursuing hobbies such as playing bridge or an instrument are less likely to lose their mental abilities over time compared with people who do not enjoy intellectually challenging activities. In the same thread of thought, people who are isolated socially and remain mostly within the confines of their own solitude or a limited circle of acquaintances are at increased risk for dementia later on.

Remember, though, these studies only find an association, not a definite causal effect. So it does not mean that everyone who does not like to exercise, read, or socialize will develop Alzheimer's disease. Humans are unique in that no two individuals are exactly the same. Even identical twins will have different personalities and interests, and lead different lives. Just because one may prefer to spend time alone rather than attending a party, or stay indoors watching television rather than going out jogging, does not mean that one is doomed to develop Alzheimer's disease. The studies show that people who stay active physically, mentally, and socially are less likely to have memory problems or develop dementia later in life. Plus, maintaining these lifestyle factors is not only beneficial for brain health but for overall health as well.

## OTHER RISK FACTORS

Besides the risk factors discussed thus far, numerous other predictors have been proposed as potential risk factors for Alzheimer's disease. Some examples include alcohol, smoking, diet, estrogen, and homocysteine. We know that excessive alcohol can lead to a type of dementia called alcoholic dementia. Some studies have looked at people with the apo-E genotype and the effects of alcohol intake, but the results have been mixed and inconclusive. The relationship between smoking and Alzheimer's disease has also been studied, but again, the results are conflicting.

Numerous dietary factors such as fat intake and certain vitamins have also been investigated. A diet high in saturated or transunsaturated ("trans-fat"), commonly found in processed and fried foods, and low in non-hydrogenated unsaturated fats, such as in fish or nuts, is known to be bad for the heart and overall health. Some reports have suggested a possible link to Alzheimer's disease, but the data is mixed. With the information currently available, no conclusion can be drawn about dietary fat intake and the risks of Alzheimer's disease. Similarly, researchers have also looked at the roles of vitamins, such as B6, B12, C, E, and folate, but more in the setting of whether higher intake of these vitamins can lower the risk of Alzheimer's disease. Again, the data is mixed.

Hormone replacement therapy, or estrogen replacement, used to be commonly given to middle-aged women undergoing menopause. At one point, hormone replacement therapy was thought to be possibly protective from dementia. Animal studies have found estrogen to enhance the cholinergic and glutamate systems, which are neurotransmitter systems important in learning and memory (Gazzaley 1996). However, the current thinking is that taking estrogen long-term can be a risk factor for dementia in older women (Rapp 2003).

Homocysteine is an amino acid found in the blood. When the homocysteine level is too high, it is associated with a higher risk of heart disease and stroke. But the data on whether it is a risk factor for Alzheimer's disease is uncertain. In addition to the potential risk factors discussed thus far, numerous others have been proposed, but none have really panned out.

As you can see, the common thread among the various risk factors that we have discussed is that they are just that—risk factors. We cannot make a definitive causal relationship. But based on the studies done thus far, some are stronger risk factors than others. Age, family history, and genetic predisposition are the biggest risk factors for Alzheimer's disease. Head injury, vascular disease, and lifestyle may also play a role. A positive association exists but to what degree and what the underlying mechanisms are is unclear. The brain is an intricate and complicated organ. What causes Alzheimer's disease to develop remains to be investigated and better understood.

# 3

# What Are the Signs of
# Alzheimer's Disease?

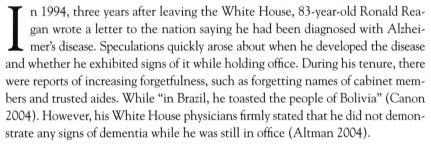

In 1994, three years after leaving the White House, 83-year-old Ronald Reagan wrote a letter to the nation saying he had been diagnosed with Alzheimer's disease. Speculations quickly arose about when he developed the disease and whether he exhibited signs of it while holding office. During his tenure, there were reports of increasing forgetfulness, such as forgetting names of cabinet members and trusted aides. While "in Brazil, he toasted the people of Bolivia" (Canon 2004). However, his White House physicians firmly stated that he did not demonstrate any signs of dementia while he was still in office (Altman 2004).

The distinction between forgetfulness as part of normal aging and memory loss in dementia is not always clear-cut. A lot of times, it is difficult to differentiate between the two during the early stages of Alzheimer's disease. This is especially true when no one is looking out for the changes. Even when someone is being closely monitored by a physician, as President Reagan was, the changes can be subtle and easily missed. And patients can be good at hiding the early signs, which are frequently dismissed as an unavoidable part of growing older. Let's look at some of the common signs of Alzheimer's disease and also try to differentiate between what is considered "normal" aging and what is not.

## MEMORY LOSS

*Dr. Brown is a well-respected physics professor who has taught at a world-renowned university for decades. His lively lectures are even broadcast on the Internet and are a big hit with students everywhere. Over the past few months, however, his students have noticed a change in him. He frequently repeats himself and makes the same statement over and over again. He often stops in the middle of class to ask questions, as he usually does to engage the students. However, he is asking the same question each time, even though it was just answered a few minutes ago. He is calling long-time students by the wrong names. His students have also shown up for scheduled office hours and found his office empty. Everyone is puzzled by the change in him.*

Many people worry about losing their memory as they get older. Memory loss is one of the most worrisome aspects of aging, due to fears of developing dementia. Memory loss is also one of the most common complaints about growing older. It is quite frustrating when you cannot recall information as quickly as when you were younger. Some people take it in stride and accept it as part of becoming older. In our society, increased absentmindedness is a widely accepted stereotype of aging. When was the last time you heard someone joke about "a senior moment" when forgetting his glasses are sitting on top of his head, after turning the house upside down looking for them? Or heard someone crack a joke about "getting senile" after finding his missing car keys in his pockets?

As one ages, occasional forgetfulness would not be unexpected. Everyone has probably experienced the frustrations of "mental blocks" at some point, where you have difficulty recalling a certain fact, such as the name to a familiar tune. But later on, when the information is no longer needed, the name of the song comes to mind out of the blue. With the aging brain, one may also need a little more time to commit new information to memory, such as learning the names of new acquaintances or remembering new phone numbers. Similarly, one may need to use a calendar to mark down appointments or to keep track of birthdays and anniversaries, when one did not need to in the past.

The big question that is frequently asked is when does forgetfulness turn into something more serious? There is no distinct boundary that separates normal age-related decline from the more serious changes in dementia that necessitate a medical evaluation. The key thing to keep in mind is that if these changes start to affect daily functioning, then this should warrant further investigation. Daily functioning is the ability to carry out the everyday tasks that are necessary to live independently, such as showering, getting dressed, or eating. Occasional forgetfulness may be normal and happens to everybody, but if it becomes more frequent and noticeable, then concern should be raised, as in Dr. Brown's case.

In Alzheimer's disease, individuals will frequently have difficulty with short-term memory. They tend to forget recent experiences quickly, such as conversations. They may forget that they have paid a bill already, and pay it again, or forget about it altogether. Family members start to notice when their loved one repeats herself or repeatedly asks questions that have already been answered several times. This is especially frustrating for spouses or children of people with dementia, having to answer the same question over and over again. Their spouses may find unpaid bills or unbalanced checkbooks when they have been doing this without difficulty for their whole adult life. They may become disheveled and wear the same dirty, wrinkled clothing daily when they have been careful with their appearances most of their lives. These are signs of memory loss in dementia.

Due to memory loss, people with Alzheimer's disease frequently misplace things. It is normal to misplace a purse or keys once in a while, only to find it sitting exactly where it was left. Even though this may happen more frequently to some people than others, it does not necessarily need to cause concern. In Alzheimer's disease, objects often become misplaced to the point where family members start getting worried. The missing items can also turn up in unexpected places. Purses have turned up in the dryer, and sweaters have been found in the kitchen cabinets. Sometimes the person can get very upset over misplaced items and even accuse loved ones of stealing. The odd locations of misplaced items can make them a challenge to locate.

As Alzheimer's disease progresses, the affected person will have progressively more difficulty with learning new information and storing it in memory. This can become quite apparent when, despite his attempts to brush off the memory loss as mere forgetfulness, the memory lapses start affecting his daily routines. Look at Dr. Brown, who forgot about weekly meetings with his students, which he has had every Tuesday for years. The person may get lost walking home. He may forget about the pot of chili simmering on the stovetop and run out for groceries. These instances of memory loss are not normal. They are common examples given by family members of patients with Alzheimer's disease, which usually concern them enough to seek out a physician.

The subtle memory changes in the early stages of dementia are often difficult to detect. Even as memory deteriorates, the changes are usually slow, which can make it tough for immediate family members to appreciate early on. Close family members will frequently comment on how despite short-term memory problems, the loved one is as sharp as a tack when it comes to recalling events in the distant past. This may be true early on, but as the dementia progresses the long-term memory starts to fade as well. But early on in the course of Alzheimer's disease, it is typically the short-term memory loss that is one of the first signs of dementia.

## LANGUAGE PROBLEMS

One noticeable slip during Ronald Reagan's presidency occurred during a highly publicized meeting with the Japanese prime minister. He introduced then Vice President Bush as "Prime Minister Bush" more than once, much to the chagrin of his aides (Thomas 1984). President Reagan's word slip may have been a simple mistake, or it may have heralded warning signs of dementia.

All of us at some point have had mishaps with using the wrong word, such as calling a spoon a fork, or using she instead of he when referring to a man. In normal aging, occasional difficulties with finding the right word can occur. Some people may have more difficulty than others, especially for those who are not native English speakers. There is no absolute distinction between age-related changes and abnormal changes seen in dementia. However, concern should be raised when the occasional trouble with word finding or word usage turns into frequent speech and language problems. Difficulty with names and word-finding becomes increasingly pronounced as Alzheimer's disease progresses.

In the early stages of dementia, the patient may struggle with recalling commonly used words or phrases. Typically, it is not alarming, and the patient is able to find an alternate word. However, as the disease progresses, it becomes more difficult to draw from the memory reserve. The patient will frequently describe the object or circumvent the topic if they are having difficulty. For example, he may say "that thing you eat with" if unable to remember a fork, or "that thing you use to clean your teeth" if referring to a toothbrush. Sometimes, the person may not be able to describe the object at all, and try to change the conversation. Or he may try to substitute with a word that makes the sentence nonsensical. Furthermore, these language problems can become pronounced in the person's writing. His letters and e-mails may start not making sense or sound incoherent.

Problems with communication frequently arise. The person may start having difficulty following conversation as he is having trouble understanding others. It can be especially frustrating when the person has trouble expressing himself and making himself understood. Being able to carry on conversations and communicate with others is an important part of daily living. It allows an individual to express his needs to others, whether it be help with something or a question. Language also allows one to convey emotions. Imagine what it would be like if you were having a toothache but could not find the right words to relay your pain. With the loss of language and speech abilities, communication with others becomes a struggle.

In later stages of Alzheimer's disease, when memory loss becomes more pronounced, the language deficits also become more noticeable. When asked specifically to recall or name certain objects, a common response may be "umm . . . you know . . . that thing." Among those who speak English as a second language, it is not uncommon for them to revert back to speaking their native language. The language loss eventually affects the person's ability to carry on a conversation, at first in a meaningful way, and toward the end, altogether. In the final stages of dementia, the individual often becomes mute, completely losing his ability to talk.

When trying to detect Alzheimer's disease as early as possible, language difficulties can be noticeable early on. Although subtle changes can be missed initially, as the dementia progresses, word-finding problems become evident in daily conversation. Persons will forget how use to certain nouns or verbs appropriately, and their speech and writing become affected.

## DISORIENTATION

*Mrs. Smith has been retired as a secretary for the CEO of a Fortune 500 company for many years. She was always proud of her ability to juggle her boss's busy schedule without fail. She never even relied on a calendar to remember her own appointments. Recently, on several occasions, her hairdresser and dentist have sent notices for missed appointments. Once, she showed up for her doctor's appointment a month early. Her daughter became worried when she missed her grandson's birthday party this year. Mrs. Smith has never forgotten one of her grandchildren's birthday before.*

Disorientation, or losing one's sense of position or time, is a common sign of Alzheimer's disease. As you can imagine, losing one's memory and not being able to form new memory makes it more difficult to keep track of time or place. When a person gets older, it is not unusual for him or her to occasionally forget why they entered the room or confuse the days of the week. The correct answer will usually come to mind later, or a quick glance at the calendar is a sufficient reminder.

In dementia, however, disorientation occurs more frequently and becomes conspicuous as the disease progresses. In Mrs. Smith's case, she started missing important appointments and birthdays due to difficulty with keeping track of dates. Having trouble judging the passage of time is also a common occurrence. In one instance, Mrs. Smith started to put on her coat to leave 10 minutes after arriving at her daughter's house because she forgot that she just got there. Another time, she woke up from a nap in the afternoon and started getting ready for work, forgetting that she has not worked in years and confusing the time of the day.

With disease progression, the changes become more serious. She may go out for a walk and forget where she is or how to get home. She may get lost driving around the neighborhood that she has lived in her whole life and have to call one of her children to get directions home. She may start confusing day and night, and mistakenly take medications twice. Or start preparing dinner in the middle of the night thinking it is suppertime. These are some examples of disorientation that commonly occur in Alzheimer's disease. Over time, the disorientation becomes impossible to hide or compensate for.

## DIFFICULTY WITH FAMILIAR TASKS

*Ever since he was a young boy, Mr. Williams has loved building airplane models. Recently, however, his wife noticed that he is not spending as much time as he used to working on his airplanes. One day, she walked by and saw him struggling with his tools. The half-finished models on the counter were put together haphazardly, a stark contrast to the beautiful airplanes that he made before which line the wall.*

As we go about our daily lives, we perform the same tasks over and over again without thinking about it. It becomes second nature to brush our teeth, button a shirt, or tie our shoes. Many people learn skills such as operating a can opener, using the television remote, or typing on a computer until these skills become effortless. In Mr. Williams's case, building airplane models was second nature from years of experience. As a person gets older, it is not uncommon to have occasional lapses in memory, such as forgetting how to set the DVD player, but this knowledge usually quickly returns. With Alzheimer's disease, these memory lapses become more frequent and noticeable as time goes on.

In someone with Alzheimer's disease, common tasks that are frequently taken for granted become challenging to perform. The person may forget what a familiar object is used for and look confused when handed a comb. He may not know what to do when handed a pencil. He may also forget steps to common tasks, such as the steps involved in brushing teeth or preparing a meal. In the early stages, if the person is still working, co-workers may notice some difficulty with performing routine tasks at work. A mechanic may start having difficulty with changing tires. Family members may become aware of something awry when bills go unpaid and checkbooks are unbalanced. Someone who has driven a car for decades may start having difficulty in the driver's seat, such as starting the car or backing the car out of the driveway.

Problems with familiar tasks can be compounded by loss of coordination. As different parts of the brain are affected by dementia, the person finds himself not being able to use his hands and feet as he would like when performing mundane tasks. He may comprehend what he wants to do, such as button a shirt, but the message is not relayed from his brain to his fingers. The loss of coordination makes it difficult to carry out routine tasks.

Initially, the individual may try to mask these deficits by avoiding activities that he is having trouble with, such as wearing shoes without shoe laces or wearing a pullover shirt so as to avoid grappling with buttons. He may stop calling friends because he is having trouble with dialing the telephone. He may order a hamburger instead of his favorite steak at a restaurant to avoid having to use forks and knives. However, as Alzheimer's disease progresses, these difficulties with familiar tasks become harder to hide because they will affect more and more skills. It becomes particularly evident to loved ones when problems with everyday activities arise. A messy house belonging to someone who has always been tidy is hard to miss. Malodorous hair and dirty clothing are not easy to camouflage, and can indicate struggles with familiar tasks. Thus, increasing difficulty with everyday chores can be a sign of Alzheimer's disease.

## PERSONALITY CHANGES

*Mr. McDonald is worried about his wife of 50 years. He cannot figure out why she has changed so drastically over the last few years. She used to be a gentle, loving woman who enjoyed going out shopping and dining with him. These days, he cannot convince her to leave the house. She prefers to sit at home all day. She also snaps at him frequently and becomes angry over little things. She used to love gardening, but has not stepped into her vegetable garden for almost a year. He is frustrated and does not know what to do.*

In addition to memory loss, Mr. McDonald's wife was exhibiting signs of personality changes that frequently occur in Alzheimer's disease. A person's temperament may change somewhat with aging but typically remains relatively stable throughout life. It is abnormal to have personality changes that are noticeable and worrisome to family members. Although the initial changes in early dementia can be subtle and easily brushed off, as the personality changes become more frequent and more noticeable, it frequently causes distress to close family members.

It can be troublesome to family members when a diagnosis has not been made, and they are trying to cope with the personality changes. Even after the diagnosis, it does not always get easier dealing with the personality changes. While understanding that these changes are unintentional and part of the disease process, being on the receiving end of sharp remarks or verbal attacks can still be quite hurtful. Even after Mr. McDonald learned that the changes in his wife's behavior were due to Alzheimer's disease, he still found it difficult not to react to his wife's verbal barrages in a personal way. He could not help feeling hurt.

Personality changes in dementia vary from person to person. The affected individuals often do not recognize the changes in themselves and resist help from concerned loved ones. A previously gregarious, outgoing person may withdraw from social interactions and become reticent. She may no longer seem interested in doing previous hobbies, such as going out with friends or watching movies. Some people with dementia can become suspicious and fearful for no apparent reason. It is not uncommon for a person with dementia to accuse family members of stealing money or personal objects. She may become afraid that someone is "coming after her" and become distrustful of everyone. These are some examples of personality changes. Everyone is unique, and frequently it is close family members and friends who notice the subtle changes first. Although personality changes can be a sign of Alzheimer's disease, there may other underlying causes as well. So an assessment by a physician is important. Some components of the assessment will be discussed later.

## MOOD AND BEHAVIOR CHANGES

As we go about our daily lives, our emotions can fluctuate throughout the course of the day. Usually, it is in reaction to certain events or interactions with others. On any given day, you may feel happy about receiving a good grade on a test, or be excited about an upcoming trip. The next day, you may become sad about a grandparent's illness. Our emotions enrich our experiences throughout daily life. It is normal to experience the whole spectrum of feelings over time, but most people are usually in a happy medium. You can feel grumpy or moody one day, but it usually passes quickly.

In Alzheimer's disease, the mood swings can be rapid and quite unexpected. Frequently, the emotions change for reasons that others cannot comprehend, and the affected individual has difficulty expressing what he is feeling. In Mr. McDonald's case, his wife would lash out at him for little things that never used to faze her. One morning, she became angry at him for making oatmeal for breakfast, when it turned out she was hoping for something else but could not remember the name for it. Mr. McDonald's wife would also at times burst into tears without instigating factors. He felt helpless as his wife's moods swung like a pendulum without clear cause.

In addition to alterations in mood, another early sign of early Alzheimer's disease is loss of initiative. It is normal to occasionally not feel like doing anything except be a couch potato. However, it is not normal to feel like this all the time. Mr. McDonald's wife used to be a social butterfly who enjoyed planning outings with friends and family. Over the past few years, she gradually lost interest in contacting friends and frequently had to be cajoled to participate in family get-togethers. Eventually, she could be barely convinced to do anything other than sit at home. Even her grandchildren could not persuade her to play with them.

To have initiative is to take action, to be eager to start a project or to do something. To lose initiative is to become indifferent and apathetic. Family members usually start to notice when a person with Alzheimer's disease loses interest in their usual activities and hobbies, as in Mrs. McDonald's case. Some people may sleep more and not want to get out of bed. Loss of initiative can also come out in the form of poor grooming. Someone who has always been a meticulous dresser may start appearing unkempt. Lack of initiative can also present as weight loss. A person living alone may lose the desire to go grocery shop and prepare meals, and, as a result, lose weight. Thus, loss of initiative can be a sign of Alzheimer's disease.

## POOR JUDGMENT

Mr. McDonald is also concerned about his wife's judgment. She has always been the responsible one in their relationship. She paid their bills on time and made sure their house was in tip-top shape. This is no longer the case. One day, he discovered that they didn't have enough money to pay the utilities. It turned out she had given large sums of money to charities that solicit donations in the mail. He now manages their finances. Another time, he found her scrubbing the bathtub with a toothbrush, when the scrubbing pad was sitting in plain sight. Mr. McDonald has also found his wife wearing sweaters in the middle of summer, and ready to walk outside in slippers and a T-shirt during a snowstorm. These are some examples of decreased judgment that is not part of normal aging.

Judgment is the ability to make a decision or form an opinion with common sense and in a logical manner. Basically, having sound judgment is to have good sense. There is a common saying that "to get older is to get wiser." The hope is that with the experiences and knowledge accumulated over a lifetime, one's judgment improves with aging. Of course, no one is perfect. It is normal to make questionable judgments once in awhile that has others scratching their heads. However, when bad decisions are made frequently or quite out of norm, then it should raise a red flag.

Frequently, persons with Alzheimer's disease do not see anything wrong with their decision-making. This often comes up when the topic turns to driving. If the affected person's memory loss and decreased thinking abilities have progressed, both physicians and family members become concerned about his driving abilities. The issue of elderly drivers has been in the media spotlight quite a bit, especially when elderly drivers are involved in tragic car accidents. If there is a question of memory impairment, then it raises even greater concern. Driving requires concentration and sound judgment. One needs to be able to react quickly and decisively to ever changing road conditions. One bad decision can lead to an accident. In Alzheimer's disease, judgment is impaired and the patient frequently is unable to recognize it. The lack of insight, or awareness, is also part of the dementia process. It can be frustrating for both the patient and the family members.

## ABSTRACT THINKING

*Mrs. Green's son had attributed his mother's increasing forgetfulness to simply "getting older" until one day when he received a call from his mother. She was at the train station in another town. After her weekly visit with a friend, she could not figure out an alternate train route to take when her usual train was canceled. Mrs. Green was also an avid cook. She loved to watch cooking shows and try new recipes from magazines. Over Thanksgiving, however, her children noticed that her usually delicious dishes tasted odd and realized she had trouble following the recipes. She was confusing teaspoons with tablespoons, and mixing up the various cup measurements.*

Abstract thinking involves thinking in conceptual or theoretical terms. It requires the ability to visualize or think about something without it being physically available. Recall the first time you learned about Newton's apple and the concept of gravity. It is a force that we know about but cannot see or feel. For centuries, the world was thought to be flat. When explorers started postulating that the world was actually round, they were met with great doubt. Abstract thinking requires the brain to visualize the world as round, even though when we are walking or driving, it feels like the earth is flat.

Abstract thinking is important in many aspects of daily life. Figuring out the sale price of an item at 20 percent off while shopping requires performing mental calculations. When your friend gives you directions to her house, it requires visualizing the roads and signs in your head. As one ages, it can be normal to have mild difficulties with filling out the annual tax returns, which can be quite complicated, or struggle a little with balancing the checkbook. In Alzheimer's disease, the impairment is much more significant.

When do problems with abstract thinking become concerning? Simple calculations, such as counting, can become challenging. The various numbers may lose meaning and become jumbled up. The individual may have trouble counting utensils when asked to set the dinner table for eight people. One store owner's family started getting concerned when he was giving out the wrong change to customers. An accountant who has always been able to do complicated arithmetic in his head started botching his clients' accounts. These are examples of problems with abstract thinking.

Difficulty with planning is common when someone has impaired abstract thinking. Mrs. Green struggled with planning out a train route to take home. When her usual train was unavailable, she needed to study the route map and plan a different course, which she was unable to do. Using public transportation is a part of many people's daily routine. Taking the bus to work requires planning out the bus routes in advance, as does riding the subway. This necessitates being able to think conceptually. When someone shows signs of impaired abstract thinking, the ability to plan out daily activities becomes affected.

The signs of Alzheimer's disease are quite varied. Patients are frequently brought in by family members to the doctor's office with different stories relating to dementia. These tales frequently share common themes of memory loss, language problems, and disorientation. They may also encompass personality, mood, and behavior changes. Decreased judgment and abstract thinking are often evident. The signs of dementia are not always obvious, especially in the early stages, where the changes are at times missed or brushed off as merely normal signs of aging. Even the affected person may be reluctant to acknowledge the changes, and instead, choose to ignore the signs. Frequently, the person is unaware of the changes and tries his best to compensate for them. However, as Alzheimer's disease progresses, the signs of dementia become more noticeable and harder to ignore, necessitating a medical evaluation.

# 4

# How Is Alzheimer's Disease Diagnosed?

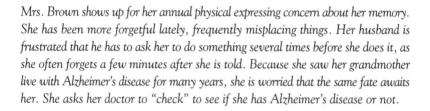

*Mrs. Brown shows up for her annual physical expressing concern about her memory. She has been more forgetful lately, frequently misplacing things. Her husband is frustrated that he has to ask her to do something several times before she does it, as she often forgets a few minutes after she is told. Because she saw her grandmother live with Alzheimer's disease for many years, she is worried that the same fate awaits her. She asks her doctor to "check" to see if she has Alzheimer's disease or not.*

It is not uncommon for patients to show up at their doctor's office requesting an evaluation for Alzheimer's disease. Due to the common perception that memory loss equates to Alzheimer's disease, many people become frightened at any signs of increased forgetfulness. Although some may simply attribute forgetfulness to growing older, hints of memory lapse can make some people nervous. Those people who have relatives or know someone who has Alzheimer's disease can be especially sensitive to any trouble remembering things and seek out medical evaluation quickly. A more common scenario involves worried spouses or children accompanying a loved one who comes grudgingly for assessment. No matter what the reason or motivation is for requesting a possible diagnosis of Alzheimer's disease, the initial approach is standard in most cases.

Definitive diagnosis of Alzheimer's disease requires examining brain tissue under the microscope, like what Dr. Alzheimer did for Auguste D. Of course, this is rarely possible in real life. Not many people would agree to have a piece of brain tissue extracted solely for a diagnosis. In a few cases, people may agree to donate their brains to research after death, thereby giving the opportunity to confirm the diagnosis. However, for the most part, Alzheimer's disease is diagnosed clinically. This means that the diagnosis is based on a doctor's assessment after compiling all the facts. When we say someone has Alzheimer's disease, it should be prefaced with "probable" or "possible" because definitive diagnosis is difficult to ascertain without actual examination of brain tissue.

The diagnosis of Alzheimer's disease involves several steps. These steps are essentially the same as for most types of dementia. There are characteristic features of Alzheimer's disease that distinguish its diagnosis from other types of dementia. Nonetheless, sometimes it is difficult to separate Alzheimer's disease from other types of dementia, as no two patients exhibit the exact same symptoms. Occasionally, someone will have atypical symptoms of Alzheimer's disease, making the diagnosis challenging. One of the main goals of the diagnostic process is identifying those medical conditions that can mimic the signs of dementia and can be potentially reversed. It is also important to arrive at a correct diagnosis in order to administer appropriate treatment. A missed or misdiagnosis can have serious implications for the individual.

The initial step in diagnosing Alzheimer's disease involves an office evaluation by a health care professional. This is where family members, or the patient himself, express their concerns to the physician. The doctor uses this opportunity to obtain a thorough history and gather all the necessary information on the events leading up to the office visit. A physical examination will follow. In addition to the physical exam, a general mental exam is also performed, which involves specific questions used to evaluate the person's mental abilities.

After the initial history taking and physical and mental exam, if Alzheimer's disease is suspected, the next step involves more specific tests. Blood tests are typically obtained. The main goal of these blood tests is to rule out other medical problems that may mimic the signs of dementia. Neuropsychologic testing is also done in most cases. It consists of a series of mental tasks to evaluate the various cognitive domains, such as memory, concentration, and language skills. The final piece of the diagnostic process typically involves head imaging, or taking scans of the brain.

Once all the information has been collected, the physician will evaluate the data as a whole and determine whether the person meets criteria for Alzheimer's disease. This process may take several office visits to complete. Because brain biopsy is rarely feasible, or desirable, the diagnosis of probable Alzheimer's disease is based on certain diagnostic criteria. These criteria are based on guidelines put out by various panels of expert physicians. Ultimately, however, the diagnosis is based on the doctor's clinical judgment.

## DIAGNOSTIC CRITERIA

Before going into detail about the various steps involved in diagnosing Alzheimer's disease, let's briefly discuss the diagnostic criteria. Diagnostic criteria refers to a set of reference points or benchmarks that must be met in order to make a positive diagnosis. It is important to understand what the criteria are, as these are the important things that the physician keeps in mind when performing the evaluation. Part of the assessment involves delving into the person's symptoms and seeing which criteria are met.

Several frameworks have been proposed for diagnosing probable Alzheimer's disease. Of these, two are mostly commonly used. One is established by the National Institute of Neurological and Communicative Disorders and Stroke and the Alzheimer's Disease and Related Disorders Association (NINCDS-ADRDA) (McKhann 1984). Do not worry about trying to remember the very long name of this organization. You just need to be aware of the initials, as they are frequently cited in publications that discuss diagnosing Alzheimer's disease. Another commonly used criterion for diagnosing Alzheimer's disease is put forth by the American Psychiatric Association in their *Diagnostic and Statistical Manual of Mental Disorders, Fourth Edition,* or DSM-IV for short (American Psychiatric Association 2000). The DSM-IV provides diagnostic criteria for mental disorders. Its guidelines are widely used by psychiatrists and health providers to aid in making diagnoses related to mental illnesses.

The criteria set out by both organizations are quite similar. First and foremost is the presence of memory impairment. It is not enough for the person to simply complain about memory loss. The memory impairment should be evident in clinical evaluation by the physician, as well as through objective measurements using memory assessment tools.

In addition to memory loss, the person should have a decline in two or more areas of cognition, or mental abilities. These four cognitive domains include aphasia, apraxia, agnosia, and disturbance in executive functioning. Aphasia refers to difficulty with speaking or understanding spoken language (phasia in Greek means "utterance," so a-phasia is "without utterance"). A person with aphasia may speak in broken sentences or have difficulty following a conversation. Apraxia (praxia means "action" in Greek) is a loss of the ability to carry out learned, purposeful movements. Examples of apraxia include difficulty with familiar activities such as writing or tying shoe laces. Agnosia ("ignorance" in Greek) is not being able to recognize familiar objects, persons, or sounds. For instance, a formerly avid tennis player may not know what to do when he is handed a racket. Executive function refers to an individual's ability to organize, carry out thoughts and activities, prioritize tasks and make decisions. Common tasks that we frequently take for granted, such as picking up the telephone and ordering pizza delivery, involve planning that may become too complicated for someone with dementia. Thus, a diagnosis of Alzheimer's disease requires impairment in at least two out of these four areas.

However, it is not enough to just have memory loss and problems with cognitive abilities. These deficits must be significant enough to cause a marked decline in the person's daily functioning, either at home or at work. A person can have some memory and cognitive problems, but if the disturbance does not affect that individual's day-to-day functioning, then it is called mild cognitive impairment. On a continuum between normal age-related memory changes and dementia, this sits between the two ends of the spectrum. It is a condition that poses increased risk for eventually developing dementia, although not everyone progresses to it (Fischer 2007). When a person experiences a significant decline in daily performance as a result of memory and cognitive decline, then it can be considered dementia. Alzheimer's disease is the most common type of dementia.

Once the memory and cognitive deficits have been determined to have caused a meaningful deterioration in daily functioning, there are several more steps to confirm the diagnosis of probable Alzheimer's disease. First, it must be determined that the course of the decline is gradual and continual. If someone comes in and says he lost his memory last week but regained it by the weekend, then it is unlikely to be dementia. Or if a person without any warning signs suddenly cannot recognize her husband, then it is less likely to be dementia. The more typical scenario involves someone who started having problems with short-term memory a few years ago, which has gotten worse recently and is now affecting his or her job performance. Another example is someone who becomes increasingly absent-minded, to the point where her husband found a missing check in the freezer. Thus, one of the requirements for diagnosing Alzheimer's disease is that the mental decline be gradual and continual.

Lastly, an important aspect of the diagnostic process is to make sure that the memory changes are not caused by other medical or mental illnesses. There are some medical conditions that can mimic the signs of dementia. It is critical to ensure that there are no other plausible explanations for the mental decline. This is accomplished by eliciting a thorough medical history from the patient. It also includes a physical examination by the physician. Furthermore, laboratory tests and imaging studies are routinely performed. Neuropsychological testing, or detailed memory and cognitive tests, can be helpful as well. It is also vital to ascertain that the memory and cognitive changes are not due to delirium, which is a temporary disturbance in consciousness. We will discuss these tests and evaluations in more detail shortly.

Let's briefly summarize the diagnostic criteria for Alzheimer's disease. A person should have memory loss and dysfunction in at least two of the four cognitive areas: aphasia, apraxia, agnosia, and executive function. The memory and cognitive deficits should be significant enough to cause a noticeable decline in everyday functioning. The decline should be gradual and persistent. It should not be due to a transient alternation in consciousness. Other medical or psychiatric illnesses should not be responsible for these changes.

One might wonder how accurate these diagnostic criteria are. After all, we are only able to diagnose probable Alzheimer's disease clinically. An absolute diagnosis requires examination of brain tissue for amyloid plaques and neurofibrillary tangles, which is rarely possible. Several studies have tried to answer this question. Dementia researchers have examined donated brains, and in one study, found an 87 percent accuracy rate when the NINCDS-ADRDA criterion was used (Gearing 1995). This means that when NINCDS-ADRDA criterion was used to diagnose Alzheimer's disease and the person's brain tissues were later examined after death, it was correct 87 percent of the time in diagnosing Alzheimer's disease. Studies looking at brain tissues of Alzheimer's patients diagnosed using the DSM-IV criterion have found similar accuracy rates (Phung 2007). This suggests that our ability to clinically diagnose Alzheimer's disease is fairly accurate but not perfect. So errors in diagnosis can occur. Let's turn now to the diagnostic process in detail.

## HISTORY AND PHYSICAL

A "history and physical" are common medical term used to describe the typical doctor's visit. The first part of the visit involves the patient describing his ailment and the physician asking specific questions to elicit details on the problems at hand. The latter portion is spent performing a physical examination. A lot of information can be gathered through a good history and physical. In fact, clinical information obtained from the history and physical is often enough to lead to a probable diagnosis for many illnesses.

### History

*History of Present Illness*

During the initial history intake, the patient has the opportunity to explain his concerns. In Alzheimer's disease, the chief complaints are typically about memory loss or difficulty with mental tasks. It is often helpful, and even critical, to have family members or close friends provide additional information. It is not uncommon for individuals with Alzheimer's disease to be unaware of their decline or refuse to acknowledge it. "There's nothing wrong with me!" is a common assertion made by indignant patients who are brought in unwillingly by concerned loved ones. The family members will often have noticed the signs of Alzheimer's disease and seen how it has affected the person's daily functioning. Thus, information provided by family members is extremely valuable in the diagnostic process.

After the patient or relative has had a chance to describe her concerns, the physician will ask targeted questions to collect specific details regarding cognitive and memory impairment. These questions are aimed at trying to determine whether the reported symptoms are consistent with dementia or due to other medical problems. The physician will also be mindful of the diagnostic criteria for Alzheimer's disease and ask questions to see if the person exhibits deficits in any of the cognitive domains other than memory loss. There is no specific checklist of questions asked by every clinician during an encounter like this. Because of the variety of symptoms, the questions are usually tailored to the individual case. But they are similar in that they are asked with the intent of ruling out other medical diagnoses as well as trying to apply the diagnostic criteria for Alzheimer's disease.

### Past Medical History

The history portion of the visit also involves obtaining a thorough understanding of the medical problems of the individual, or the "past medical history." The physician asks about previously diagnosed medical problems and hospitalizations, keeping an eye out for the risk factors for Alzheimer's disease that were discussed earlier. Thus, the person is often asked about whether he has high blood pressure, high cholesterol, or diabetes. Whether he has had a stroke or head injury is also of interest. The person is also asked about prior surgeries or medical procedures, especially if they involved the brain. Certain portions of the brain may have been removed or manipulated, thereby affecting mental abilities. Whether the person has a history of depression or other mental illnesses is important information as well. A careful scrutiny of the individual's past medical history can provide useful information.

### Medications

The next part of the history taking is a review of the medications that the individual is taking. This is an important aspect of the diagnostic process for Alzheimer's disease. All medications can cause potential side effects, no matter if they are prescribed by a doctor or purchased over the counter from the local drug store. A side effect is an undesirable effect caused by a medication in addition to its intended use. Because everyone's body is different, no single person reacts to a drug in the same manner. Thus, the adverse reactions associated with a medication can range from mild discomfort to serious complications resulting in death. The elderly, in particular, are more susceptible to undesirable side effects due to age-related changes to the body. Older adults are also more likely to take multiple medications, which can interact with each other and cause undesirable effects on the body.

Reviewing medications as part of the evaluation for Alzheimer's disease involves looking for those drugs that can cause confusion or memory loss as a result of an unintended side effect. In some instances, removing these medications can lead to significant improvement in memory and cognition. The individual should be asked about all medications, including those prescribed by a physician, or those purchased over the counter at a drugstore, or herbal supplements obtained at health stores. Over-the-counter drugs are those readily available at local pharmacies that can be purchased without a physician's guidance. Some examples include cough syrups and pain medications such as ibuprofen. There are some nonprescription medications, such as sleeping aids, with side effects that can impair memory and thinking abilities. In terms of herbal supplements, there are countless brands and preparations available. Herbal supplements are not regulated by the U.S. Federal Drug Administration. Most have not been well studied, both in terms of their intended and untoward side effects. It is also helpful to inquire about previous medication use. Sometimes, an individual may have started taking a medication for memory prescribed by previous physicians in the past and not know that this was the reason the drug was given. This information can provide more details on the timeline of the memory deficit, as well as more clues to help in the diagnosis.

After reviewing the medications in detail, the physician will take some time to understand the individual's background better. Information about the person's social and family history will be gathered. The individual may be asked to describe his typical day, which provides information on his functional status. It also provides a sense of his level of physical activity as well as degree of social interactions.

### Social History

The social history refers to the individual's social background. He will be asked about his education level, which may influence how well he does on memory tests. Whether he is a native English speaker or has another primary language may affect his performance on the language portion of cognitive assessment. The person will also be asked to recount his occupational history. Habits such as smoking and alcohol will be queried. Someone who drinks alcohol excessively is at risk for developing memory problems, sometimes even developing a type of dementia called alcoholic dementia. A chronic smoker may be predisposed to vascular disease. The doctor will also ask about illicit drug use, such as marijuana or cocaine, which are known to blunt mental abilities.

### Family History

The individual's family history is also explored. The patient will be questioned about his family history, in particular, whether any relatives have been diagnosed with Alzheimer's disease before. Sometimes older generations, such as grandparents or great-grandparents, were noted to have memory loss but never taken to a doctor. Thus, no official diagnosis would have been made. Although a positive family history for Alzheimer's disease is not factored into the diagnostic criteria, it is a risk factor and can be helpful information, especially if there is a particularly strong family association. For example, if a person's mother and grandmother were diagnosed with Alzheimer's disease at younger ages, then it would raise greater suspicion compared to someone with a distant uncle who had it. However, that's not to say that someone without a family history is exempt, as every person should receive a complete evaluation. In addition to asking about family members with dementia, the doctor takes a family history of other illnesses as well, especially those that may manifest themselves like Alzheimer's disease, such as other types of dementia, Parkinson's disease, depression, or mental illnesses.

### Functional History

Next, a discussion about the person's daily functioning ensues, which is an important part of the history taking. Remember, one of the criteria for diagnosing probable Alzheimer's disease is demonstrating a marked decline in everyday functioning. Daily functioning is a person's ability to take care of him or herself and carry out those activities necessary to live independently. These daily activities are typically broken down into two categories.

The first is a cluster of activities that are essential to meeting daily personal needs, commonly referred to as basic Activities of Daily Living (ADL) by health professionals. This includes walking, using the toilet, bathing, grooming, dressing, and eating. These are the first skills that we all learn when growing up. Being able to manage these personal care needs throughout the day is crucial. Beyond these sets of skills are additional activities that indicate a higher level of functioning, called Instrumental Activities of Daily Living (IADL). Some examples are managing money, light household chores, shopping for groceries, cooking, and using a telephone.

The physician asks about these activities to assess the individual's degree of functioning and whether there has been a marked decline. Typically, the individual will exhibit difficulties in Instrumental Activities of Daily Living early on, as these tasks are more complicated. As Alzheimer's disease progresses into the more advanced stages, the impairments will encroach upon the basic activities of daily living. Deterioration in particular skills can also give clues about the types of cognitive deficit that the individual is experiencing. For instance, problems using a telephone can indicate agnosia, not recognizing the phone or numbers, or apraxia, forgetting how to pick up the phone and dial. Thus, the functional history can provide valuable information to aid in the diagnosis of Alzheimer's disease.

**Physical Exam**

Let's now move on to the physical exam. The physical exam involves checking the individual over, as well as performing a neurologic exam that includes memory testing. This portion of the evaluation can provide a lot of information and help in making the diagnosis of Alzheimer's disease.

First, before the physician whips out her stethoscope, she observes the person. This can be done during the first handshake, and throughout the interview. Physical appearance can be quite informative. Is the person immaculately dressed? Or is he wearing mismatched socks and wrinkled clothing? Is he wrapped in a scarf and heavy coat on a sweltering day? Just observing someone's physical appearance can be revealing.

In addition to outer appearances, careful observation of the person's countenance and mannerism is a part of the physical exam. How is the person acting? Is he engaged in the conversation? Or is he slumped in the chair and not making eye contact? Is his speech making sense? Or is he not answering the questions directly, and becoming belligerent and defensive? These observations can provide important clues in the diagnosis.

*Vital Signs*

You probably recall a similar routine every time you go to the doctor's office. You have to first stand on a scale. Then a nurse will wrap a cuff around your arm and check your blood pressure. She will also measure your pulse. Sometimes she will stick a thermometer under your tongue to check your body temperature. These measurements are called vital signs. They offer information on one's overall health and basic bodily functions. Vital signs typically include temperature, blood pressure, and respiratory rate (or how fast the person is breathing). Weight is usually assessed as well. These numbers can be very helpful in the process of diagnosing probable Alzheimer's disease.

In an elderly person, unintentional weight loss can be an alarming sign. There are numerous potential explanations for weight loss, and dementia is one of them. Weight loss usually requires further medical evaluation, which can lead to other diagnoses that may have overlapping symptoms. In someone who is taking medications to control high blood pressure, seeing how well it is regulated can be informative. If the blood pressure is uncontrolled, then it may suggest that the individual is forgetting to take his medications or not taking them correctly. This would also raise concern about his ability to manage his other medical problems. The pulse, or how fast the heart is beating, can be informative as well. For someone who has an irregular heartbeat, which may be abnormally fast, taking a medication to control the heart rate is critical. But if the pulse is found to be beating too fast, then it may indicate that person is not taking his medicines properly. Thus, the vital signs offer clues in trying to reach a diagnosis for Alzheimer's disease. They are another piece of the puzzle that helps the physician put the whole picture together.

*Physical Exam*

After reviewing the vital signs and weight, the next component of the physical exam involves examining the individual from head to toe. This means that, starting from the eyes and working all the way down to the feet, the various organ systems are assessed. This is a standard physical exam that is performed in most doctors' office visits. The head, eyes, ears, nose, and throat are checked. The neck is examined and thyroid gland (which sits in the front of the neck) palpated to see if it is enlarged or tender. The clinician then listens to how well air moves through the lungs via a stethoscope placed on the back. Next, the stethoscope is placed on the chest to listen to the heart beat. The abdomen is examined with both the stethoscope and by hand. The arms, hand, legs, and feet are looked at as well. Depending on the patient's symptoms, a more detailed exam ensues, focusing on the particular complaints.

The physical examination can provide clues to other systemic illnesses that may be contributing to the memory problems. For example, if the person has decreased vision, it can exacerbate his ability to recognize familiar faces. If an individual has hearing loss, it can explain his difficulty in following conversations or why he is struggling with simple instructions. If he has missing or rotting teeth, it may cause him to stop wanting to cook or eat. In another instance, if the person has arthritis in his fingers, it can make tasks that require fine motor skills, such as buttoning a shirt or tying shoes, hard. Therefore, performing a thorough physical exam can yield valuable information when evaluating someone for Alzheimer's disease.

### Neurologic Exam

A neurologic exam is an integral part of the physical diagnosis. It is an assessment of the nervous system, consisting of several components. This includes evaluating the cranial nerves, motor and sensory systems, reflexes, coordination, gait, and mental status. These tests offer insights into the functionalities of various areas in the nervous system.

The cranial nerves are a set of nerves that relay information between the brain and the head and neck. These nerves control motor and sensory functions, such as vision, hearing, smell, taste, and facial movements. Many tests can be performed to see whether the cranial nerves are functioning normally. Some examples include checking eyesight, eye muscle movement, facial symmetry, ability to smell, and sensation in the head, face, and neck. An abnormality in one of the cranial nerve functions can indicate a breakdown anywhere in the transmission from the brain where signals are generated to the final body part receiving the signal. This can occur in conditions such as a stroke or other neurologic diseases, which may have symptoms that overlap with Alzheimer's disease.

The motor system refers to the part of the nervous system that controls movement and the muscles that it innervates. A motor exam involves observing the muscles for abnormal movements, such as twitching or tremors. Muscle strength is also evaluated in the major muscle groups, especially in the arms and legs. Weakness in any limb or on one side may signal an aberration in the motor system, which can occur in a stroke or neurologic diseases.

In addition to cranial nerve and motor exams, a sensory exam is part of the neurologic evaluation. The sensory system is the part of the nervous system that receives, processes, and sends sensory information from the body to the brain. A sensory exam involves testing different types of senses, such as pressure, pain, vibration and temperature. For example, the person may be asked to identify a warm or cold object placed on different parts of the body. Or he may need to describe the location of a vibrating tuning fork placed on his body while his eyes are closed. As with the cranial nerve and motor exams, a sensory impairment can suggest the presence of neurologic diseases and warrants further evaluation.

Gait is the manner in which a person walks. The way an individual walks can provide a lot of information about his mobility. A common assessment performed in elderly patients is the "Up and Go Test." The person is asked to stand up from a chair without using his arms for support, walk approximately 10 feet, and return to sitting in the chair without his arms. Some of things the clinician will observe are whether he has the strength to get up without using his arms, whether he is steady when he stands and walks, whether his steps are symmetrical, and how fast he walks. If the person needs to rock in the chair several times before he is able to get out of the chair, it suggests weaknesses or deconditioning in his leg muscles. If he sways or needs to hold on to something while standing, the person may have balance problems. The way the person walks, such as limping on one side or shuffling his feet, can suggest underlying medical or neurologic problems. Thus, a gait assessment is an important part of the physical exam.

The neurologic assessment is performed to evaluate the nervous system and try to detect any abnormalities or deficits. In addition to the cranial nerves and motor and sensory exams, the clinician will also check the person's reflexes and coordination. Another crucial component of the neurologic assessment is the mental status exam, which will be discussed next. Of note, any neurologic aberration on physical examination may necessitate further evaluation by a neurologist, which is a doctor specialized in the nervous system.

*Neurologic Exam: Mental Status*    Mental status tests are used to assess the individual's memory and cognitive abilities. In an initial office visit to assess memory loss, a test consisting of a short series of questions is typically given. Many cognitive tests are available to screen for dementia, and not every physician will use the same one. These memory tests were developed to try to tease out the status of the individual's memory and cognitive abilities and gauge whether they are severe enough to suggest dementia.

One of the most commonly used tests is called the Mini-Mental State Exam (MMSE) (Folstein 1975). It typically takes less than 10 minutes to complete. The test comprises a series of questions to assess a broad range of mental abilities, such as short-term memory, calculation, and language. Some of the questions include having the individual give the date and his current location, such as the state, county, and city. Short-term memory is tested by having the person learn three words and recall them in a few minutes. Writing is tested by having the person write a sentence that includes a noun and verb. The individual is also asked to identify three objects. For evaluating speech, the person is asked to repeat a phrase. Attention and calculation are assessed by having the person count backward in sevens, starting at 100 (e.g., 100, 93, 86, etc.). Points are assigned to each question or task, and a total score is tallied up. Scores below a certain cutoff are suggestive of dementia.

The MMSE is one of the most frequently used screening tools by clinicians for an initial evaluation of memory loss. Getting a low score is suggestive of dementia, but the test is not completely foolproof, especially in detecting mild Alzheimer's disease. In one study, it was able to detect dementia in 87 percent of the cases (Crum 1993). This means that the MMSE is correct in detecting dementia more than 80 percent of the time but still misses some occurrences. On the other hand, it can also falsely detect cases of dementia when the individual does not have the condition. However, these "false positives" occur in almost all types of tests. The MMSE is useful as a tool, in addition to the other aspects of the diagnostic process in evaluating someone for Alzheimer's disease. There are also other short memory tests available to screen for dementia. These tools are used to objectively measure memory loss as well as cognitive impairment.

### Delirium

Now let's touch briefly on the issue of delirium. One of the diagnostic criteria for Alzheimer's disease is to make sure the individual does not have delirium. Delirium is commonly used in everyday conversation to describe someone who is confused and agitated. One image that is frequently conjured up in historical movies is an ill woman thrashing and moaning in bed, feverish with "delirium." In medical terms, delirium refers to an acute confusional state that comes on rapidly. The affected individual will be inattentive, or have trouble focusing and paying attention. The person can alternate between acting out and being agitated, and periods of somnolence. Frequently, it is in the setting of an acute mental or physical illness. Rather than a single cause, several factors usually contribute to delirium.

When someone has delirium, he may look like he has the signs of dementia. He may not recognize family members or recall recent events and may say things that do not make any sense. However, it is important to differentiate between dementia and delirium. Delirium usually occurs acutely, compared to a slow, progressive onset in dementia. A person may be going about his life without any problems one day and become confused and agitated the next after falling ill with pneumonia. This would be more consistent with delirium rather than dementia. Furthermore, delirium is expected to resolve over time if the underlying medical conditions are treated or the "culprit" medications are removed. In Alzheimer's disease, the individual's cognition may improve, but the progressive course of dementia does not halt. These are a couple of distinctions between dementia and delirium. Sometimes, it is very difficult to distinguish between the two, as a person with dementia can also develop delirium. When trying to diagnose probable

Alzheimer's disease, one of the criteria is to ensure the memory and cognitive changes are not related to delirium.

### Depression

Another medical condition that can mimic symptoms of dementia is depression. All of us occasionally feel sad or down. When these periods of sadness become prolonged and affect daily living, it can become a medical condition called depression that needs to be treated. Some examples of depressive symptoms include poor appetite, loss of motivation, and problems with sleep. Increased forgetfulness and poor concentration can also occur. These can be mistaken for symptoms of Alzheimer's disease. Thus, screening for depression is an important part of the evaluation for Alzheimer's disease.

As with other screening tools, there are several types of questionnaires available to detect depression. The Geriatric Depression Scale (GDS) is one of the more frequently used tools. (Yesavage 1983) Because depression can appear different in the elderly compared to younger adults, this screening test was developed to detect depression in older adults. It consists of a series of questions about the person's mood. One sample question is "Do you prefer to stay at home rather than going out and doing new things?" Another question asks, "Do you feel you have more problems with memory than most?" If the individual answers positively above a certain cutoff number, then it raises suspicion about the presence of depression. This would warrant further evaluation, as well as possible referral to a psychiatrist, which is a physician specialized in treating mental disorders.

As with delirium, it is important to differentiate between dementia and depression, as these are distinct medical conditions that warrant different treatments. Due to overlapping symptoms, it can sometimes be difficult to separate depression from dementia. Depression can occur in persons with Alzheimer's disease. Furthermore, all three conditions—dementia, delirium, and depression—can occur simultaneously, which can make diagnosis especially challenging. Treating depression can result in improvement of memory and cognitive abilities. However, it is important to keep in mind that in someone with Alzheimer's disease, treating depression would not halt the progressive nature of the disease.

## LABORATORY TESTS

After performing a thorough history taking and physical exam, the next step in diagnosing Alzheimer's disease is performing laboratory tests. One of the main diagnostic criteria is to ensure the memory and cognitive decline are not secondary to, or caused by, other medical conditions. Laboratory tests, or blood tests, provide valuable information on many organ systems. Thus, blood tests allow us to detect certain medical illnesses that may be contributing to the patient's cognitive deficits.

Currently, there is no single test available to detect Alzheimer's disease. Scientists are working hard on this. There is a special genetic blood test to check for ApoE, but it is not widely used. Remember, ApoE poses increased risk for Alzheimer's disease. However, it is not diagnostic of Alzheimer's disease. Right now, this test is not widely available and is typically used in special circumstances, such as in cases of suspected early-onset Alzheimer's disease or extensive family history. For now, blood tests are mainly used to rule out potential medical conditions that can mimic dementia, especially those that can be treated and potentially reversed or improve the symptoms. For example, a urinary tract infection can cause increasing confusion in some elderly people, which improves with treating the infection.

One of the tests typically performed is a blood count, looking for white blood cells. Like soldiers protecting a country from outside threats, white blood cells are important in mounting the body's defense against infections. The level of white blood cells frequently rises when there is an infection brewing in the body, such as pneumonia or a urinary tract infection. Elderly people, in particular, are susceptible to developing delirium in the setting of an infection. Ruling out delirium is an important part of diagnosing dementia. If the number of white blood cells is abnormally elevated, it may necessitate investigating further for infections or other medical illnesses.

Red blood cells are usually included in a blood count. Red blood cells carry oxygen and nutrients to and waste products away from vital organs. A low red blood cell count is called anemia. Anemia is not known to be related to memory loss, but it can herald serious medical conditions that necessitate further evaluation.

The panel of blood tests will also include kidney function. Well-functioning kidneys are critical to maintaining overall health. Our body's waste products are mainly eliminated by the kidneys. When the kidneys become damaged and do not work as well, waste products can build up in the body. At toxic levels, the individual can become confused and disoriented, developing symptoms not unlike dementia.

In addition, electrolytes such as sodium and potassium are checked too. Electrolytes are minerals in the body that have an electric charge and are important in cell functioning. They can be found in the blood, tissue, and fluids. Many bodily functions are dependent on maintaining electrolyte balance, such as nerve, heart, and muscle function. Electrolytes are also critical in maintaining fluid balance. Dehydration, or when the body does not have enough water, can manifest as delirium in severe cases. Some electrolytes that are examined in detail include sodium, potassium, and calcium. Abnormally high or low levels of these electrolytes can be dangerous. Sodium levels, in particular, when too high or too low can cause symptoms of confusion, inattention, and fatigue. Abnormally high levels of calcium can also lead to confusion and disorientation that, if slowly progressively elevated over time, can appear similar to signs of dementia. The change in mental abilities related to aberrant calcium levels can improve markedly by correcting the calcium level.

Liver function is also evaluated as part of the panel of laboratory tests. The liver is involved in many important roles in the body, including storing nutrients, breaking down harmful substances such as alcohol and medication by-products, and removing waste products from the blood. If the liver is not working properly, these unprocessed waste products can build up in the system and cause many problems, including confusion and problems with thinking abilities in severe cases. Thus, liver function tests are routinely performed as part of the dementia assessment.

Thyroid function tests are routinely checked as a part of a dementia evaluation. The thyroid is a small gland located at the front of the neck. It secretes hormones that regulate metabolism, or how the body uses energy from food. Abnormally high or low levels of thyroid hormone can lead to problems with body temperature control, weight loss or weight gain, and poor energy level. Undersecretion of thyroid hormones, in particular, can manifest as slowed thinking, poor concentration, and problems with short-term memory. Some studies have suggested a link between Alzheimer's disease and hypothyroidism, or underactive thyroid gland, but this theory has not been confirmed and remains inconclusive. Correcting an underactive thyroid can sometimes improve memory and cognition significantly if this is the main underlying cause.

Another test that is typically ordered is one to measure vitamin B12 level. An adequate level of vitamin B12 is necessary for normal red blood cell production and nerve cell function. It is usually acquired through the diet, in particular, from meat and dairy products. Thus, people who have problems with stomach and intestine absorption are especially susceptible. Because vitamin B12 is important in maintaining normal nerve cell function, a deficiency in this vitamin can disrupt brain and nerve cell function. Vitamin B12 deficiency can manifest as poor memory, lack of energy, and other signs of dementia. Therefore, it is important to check the vitamin B12 level as part of the diagnostic process for Alzheimer's disease. Replenishing vitamin B12 in a deficient state can lead to improvements in memory.

Lastly, a test for syphilis is frequently ordered in the panel of laboratory tests. Syphilis is a primarily sexually transmitted disease caused by a bacterium called *Treponeda pallidum*. Untreated syphilis can spread throughout the body, eventually to the brain in advanced stages of the disease. Neurosyphilis ("neuro" means brain) is syphilis involvement of the brain. It may take years to manifest. Progression to such an advanced stage of the disease has become less common since penicillin became widely used to treat syphilis. The affected individual typically exhibits forgetfulness early on, which eventually progresses to memory loss and behavioral and personality changes—common symptoms that can be seen in dementia. Since the development of good treatment options for syphilis, it is now rare to see advanced stages of this disease. However, it should still be checked as some people may escape early detection of syphilis and it might be allowed to fester. Testing for syphilis is especially important in someone who presents with atypical dementia features, such as at a very young age or with acute onset of symptoms.

These are some routine blood tests commonly performed when trying to diagnose Alzheimer's disease. Based on the history and physical, additional tests may be obtained as well. Besides blood tests, urine or even spinal fluid may be evaluated depending on the circumstances. The goal of checking laboratory tests is to see if potentially reversible causes of dementia can be identified. Correcting any abnormalities may improve memory and cognition, and at times, quite significantly. However, more frequently, the test results do not show any significant abnormalities, thus pointing toward a diagnosis of probable Alzheimer's disease.

## BRAIN IMAGING

Neuroimaging, or brain imaging, is commonly performed when evaluating someone with suspected Alzheimer's disease. There are various noninvasive technologies that can take pictures of the brain and allow doctors to see the inside of the head without actually cutting it open. The purpose of brain imaging in the diagnostic process is to rule out other medical conditions that can explain the individual's symptoms. Currently, there are no specific findings on brain imaging that are synonymous with an Alzheimer's disease diagnosis. There may be characteristic findings, such as shrinkage in certain areas, that are suggestive but not diagnostic. The main use of brain imaging is to ensure there no other potential causes. Some examples are strokes, tumors (or abnormal tissue growth), bleeding, and increased brain fluid causing pressure and compression on brain tissue.

While there are various technologies available, the two most frequently used imaging modalities are CT (computed tomography) and MRI (magnetic resonance imaging) scans. CT scans, sometimes referred to as "CAT" scans, pass a series of X-ray beams through the head. It is painless and usually takes only a few minutes. It gives cross-sectional images of the brain, like taking thin slices of the brain and being able to look at each slice individually. In this way, it provides details on the various brain structures. The images used to be developed into film but are now more commonly transferred to a computer screen. Brain MRI also provides structural images of the brain by using radio waves and a magnetic field. Both CT and MRI scans have their own strengths and weaknesses, and are valuable in their own ways. MRI scans provide more detailed anatomical images and are usually preferred, but not everyone can tolerate MRI scans. It involves lying inside an enclosed tube and may not be appropriate for someone afraid of confinement. Plus, certain metals, such as a heart pacemaker, are not allowed inside an MRI scanner. Thus, the imaging modality is typically chosen based on the needs of the individual.

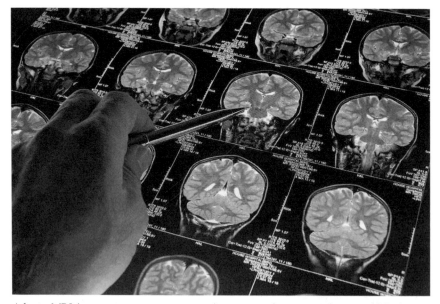

A brain MRI (magnetic resonance imaging) scan provides structural images of the brain and is used in diagnosing Alzheimer's to exclude other medical conditions that can potentially cause the person's symptoms. (iStockPhoto)

What are we looking for when brain imaging is obtained? As alluded to earlier, it is to exclude other medical conditions that can potentially cause the person's symptoms. Small blood vessel disease over time can lead to brain atrophy, or wasting away or shrinkage of brain tissue. Such changes of particular areas of the brain can lead to specific cognitive changes. For example, one type of dementia, called frontotemporal dementia, has a characteristic finding of degeneration in the frontal and temporal lobes. Another aberration that is evaluated on neuroimaging is a stroke. A stroke, or interruption of blood supply that leads to brain damage, can disrupt certain brain functions depending on the location of the injury. You have probably seen someone who has had a major stroke, where the person loses use of one side of the body and cannot speak clearly. Some strokes can result in physical impairments that are less obvious, where the only signs are memory loss or personality changes. This is why it is important to obtain head imaging when evaluating someone for Alzheimer's disease and search for other probable explanations.

As there is only so much space inside the skull, anything else, be it tissue, blood, or fluid, would compress the brain tissue. One structural abnormality that is looked for is a possible tumor, or abnormal tissue growth. Sometimes a person may bump his head without realizing it, bleeding inside the skull occurs, and a collection of blood may accumulate, thereby pressing on brain tissue. The brain has a certain amount of fluid, called cerebrospinal fluid, that plays several roles, including cushioning the brain from blows to the head and lessening the impact. When an abnormal increase in fluid occurs, it can cause pressure on the brain, thereby affecting brain function. The presence of abnormal brain tissue, blood, and fluids typically causes structural changes to the brain that can be detected on MRI or CT. These changes can alter brain function, and the individual may develop problems with memory and cognition not unlike that seen in dementia.

## NEUROPSYCHOLOGICAL TESTING

Neuropsychological testing consists of a battery of tests that evaluate a person's cognitive abilities in detail. It is not ordered for every person concerned about his memory. However, when dementia is suspected and the individual has some deficits on the screening test, such as the MMSE, then a neuropsychological test is warranted. It is also helpful when the person presents with atypical symptoms that make diagnosis a challenge.

A neuropsychological test is like an extended version of the MMSE. It is performed by a neuropsychologist, who is specially trained to administer and interpret these tests. A session can take up to two hours to complete. Some examples of cognitive abilities that are tested include memory, attention, calculation, and language. The individual may be asked to remember items, identify objects, and perform calculations. Recall that the diagnosis of Alzheimer's disease requires impairments in at least two of four cognitive domains, aphasia, apraxia, agnosia, and disturbance in executive functioning. The tasks are aimed to tease out any deficits in these areas. These tests are also trying to correlate the cognitive deficit to a structural location in the brain. After administering the test, the neuropsychologist will score and interpret the results. He or she will review the results with the physician, as well as with the patient and family members.

Neuropsychological testing is frequently used as an adjunctive tool in diagnosing Alzheimer's disease. Studies have shown it to be quite accurate in detecting dementia, although like all tests, it can miss some cases or inaccurately diagnose others. However, most of the time, neuropsychological testing is quite helpful in the diagnostic process. In terms of diagnosing Alzheimer's disease, the neuropsychological test results may conclude characteristic findings for Alzheimer's disease, such as impairments in memory and particular cognitive domains. But because some forms of dementia have overlapping features, it is not always possible to distinguish between the different types of dementia. Nonetheless, neuropsychological testing is a useful tool frequently used to aid in diagnosing Alzheimer's disease.

Definitive diagnosis of Alzheimer's disease is not always feasible as brain tissue examination is necessary. To diagnose probable Alzheimer's disease, various diagnostic criteria have been proposed, but they have similar features. It is necessary to document memory loss and cognitive impairment, while making sure other culprits are not causing the problems. The process of a history and physical, laboratory tests, brain imaging, and neuropsychological testing are intended to meet this goal. This diagnostic process can be carried out by geriatricians (doctors who specialize in the elderly), neurologists (doctors specialized in the nervous system), and geriatric psychiatrists (mental health physicians). Depending on the symptoms, one or all three may be involved in diagnosing and treating the individual.

# 5

# How Is Alzheimer's Disease Treated?

*A middle-aged woman notices that her elderly father is becoming more forgetful and withdrawn. She takes him to the doctor, who diagnoses him with Alzheimer's disease. The doctor prescribes him a "memory pill," and his memory improves markedly. The middle-aged woman stands in the doorway and watches her elderly father happily play with his grandchildren. She smiles and says she is happy to have her father back.*

This is a common scenario that is frequently portrayed in commercials for medications to treat Alzheimer's disease. But does it happen in real life?

When a diagnosis of Alzheimer's disease is made, the next question raised is usually how is it treated? Or rather, is there a cure for Alzheimer's disease? It is a grim diagnosis to receive. Even though family members probably already anticipated such a diagnosis, the news can still come as a shock. In particular, learning about the progressive nature of the disease and realizing that the mental decline will continue can be difficult to come to terms with.

The hope for any medical illness is a cure. Unfortunately, as of now, there is no cure for Alzheimer's disease. It is a complex disease without a clear cause identified yet, thus making disease prevention or cure impossible at this point. However, scientists have made great advances in understanding the disease process, and hopefully, medications to directly prevent or stop the disease are on the horizon.

Currently, the focus of treatment involves trying to delay the disease course, maintaining mental function, as well as managing the various symptoms that may arise. Managing Alzheimer's disease involves taking care of the person as a whole. It requires keeping the person physically well, socially engaged, and mentally stimulated. It also necessitates working with the caregiver to address any problems that arise as the disease progresses. Thus, unlike some diseases that simply require medications, the treatment of Alzheimer's disease involves taking care of all aspects of the individual.

The treatment of Alzheimer's disease first requires an accurate diagnosis. As discussed in the previous chapter, part of the diagnostic process is identifying key characteristics for Alzheimer's disease, and making sure the symptoms are not related to other types of dementia or illnesses. A misdiagnosis can lead to the formulation of an inappropriate treatment plan, which may be detrimental rather than helpful. Thus, it is not enough to assume a diagnosis of Alzheimer's disease, given the implications of the disease. Sometimes, individuals come to their doctor requesting treatment for Alzheimer's disease because they are convinced they have it. But it is important to perform a thorough evaluation before arriving at the diagnosis.

After a diagnosis of probable Alzheimer's disease is made, the next step is treatment. It can be considered in terms of pharmacologic and non-pharmacologic management. Pharmacology is the study or science of drugs. Thus, pharmacologic treatment is the use of medications. Several medications are currently available in the United States to treat Alzheimer's disease. These drugs are aimed at preserving the cognitive abilities for as long as possible but do not stop or reverse the disease. There are also some medications used to treat the behavioral symptoms, such as sleep or mood disturbances, but these drugs are not used exclusively in Alzheimer's disease. A non-pharmacologic approach is to manage the symptoms without using medications. This involves addressing issues such as nutrition or falls that typically occur as the disease progresses. Caregivers are also counseled on methods to handle symptoms as they arise, in order to support the individual in a safe environment and avoid acceleration in mental decline. Frequently, both pharmacologic and non-pharmacologic interventions are used concurrently in managing Alzheimer's disease, with the goal of maintaining overall health and function.

## PHARMACOLOGIC MANAGEMENT

At the present time, there are four medications approved by the U.S. Food and Drug Administration (FDA) to treat Alzheimer's disease. They may help slow down the decline of cognitive abilities but do not halt the progression of Alzheimer's disease or reverse the adverse brain changes. The medications can be categorized by their mechanism of action, or how the drug acts on the brain. Recall that neurons, or brain cells, communicate with each other via neurotransmitters. Neurotransmitters are chemical messengers that are released by neurons and carry information to intended neurons. The drugs available to treat Alzheimer's disease attempt to regulate these neurotransmitters. One class of drugs acts on the neurotransmitter acetylcholine, and the other class affects a different neurotransmitter, glutamate.

Most drugs have a generic name and many also have one or more brand names. For example, ibuprofen is the generic name for both Motrin and Advil, which are brand names. A generic drug has the same chemical equivalent, or formula, as the brand name version. It can be too confusing to keep track of different names for each medication, so after introducing the brand name, we will refer to the drugs used to treat Alzheimer's symptoms by their generic names.

## CHOLINESTERASE INHIBITORS

Cholinesterase inhibitors are currently considered the first-line treatment for Alzheimer's disease when pharmacologic management is being considered. There are four medications available under this classification of drugs called cholinesterase inhibitors. The four medications are Cognex (tacrine), Aricept (donepezil), Razadyne (galantamine), and Exelon (rivastigmine). Tacrine was the first drug approved by the FDA, but due to its harmful effects on the liver, it is rarely used anymore (Watkins 1994). The other three are prescribed more frequently. This class of drugs was developed when it was noted that individuals with Alzheimer's disease tend to have a decreased amount of a neurotransmitter called acetylcholine in the brain.

Brain cells, neurons, have a long fiber-like extension called an axon. When a neurotransmitter is released from the axon, it travels across a tiny space between the neuron, releasing it and the neuron receiving it, called a synaptic cleft. It then "docks" at specific receptors in the receiving neuron. Through this process, information is transmitted that activates a sequence of electrical impulses. In Alzheimer's disease, the production of acetylcholine appears to be reduced, which means fewer neurotransmitters are available.

As the name "inhibitor" implies, these drugs prohibit the breakdown of acetylcholine by the "cholinesterase." To put it simply, cholinesterase is an enzyme that breaks down acetylcholine. By blocking the normal action of the cholinesterase, more acetylcholine is allowed to remain within the synaptic cleft. This is believed to be the mechanism of action of cholinesterase inhibitors. Increasing the amount of acetylcholine in synapses in acetylcholine-deficient Alzheimer's patients appears to improve cognition.

Cholinesterase inhibitors are approved by the FDA for use in treating individuals with mild to moderate Alzheimer's disease. In clinical trials, which are studies that evaluate the safety and effectiveness of new drugs and treatments, these medications were shown to have a small benefit in slowing the decline of cognitive abilities (Birks 2006). This was determined by administering memory and cognitive tests before and after starting the medication. However, one concern that has been raised is how much these test scores translate to actual benefits in daily life. Thus, some studies have also measured the effect of these drugs on patients' ability to carry out activities of daily living, tasks essential to basic self-care, such as toileting and bathing. The drugs demonstrated a modest benefit in slowing the decline in such activities. There may also be a small benefit in reducing the number of behavioral disturbances (Kawas 2003). Individual response to cholinesterase inhibitors varies from individual to individual, with reports of marked improvement to a complete lack of response. Some people show a response initially, but the improvement tapers off later on. Thus, before starting the medication, it is important to discuss the risks and expected benefits in detail with the patient and family members. The goal of using these medications in treating Alzheimer's disease is to delay the decline for as long as possible, in order to help the affected individual maintain as much of his or her cognitive abilities as possible. Unfortunately, these drugs do no stop or reverse the disease process.

All three of the commonly used drugs, donepezil, galantamine, and rivastigmine, work essentially the same way, and clinical trials have shown all three of them to be equally effective. Their side effects, or unwanted response in addition to the intended effects, are also similar. Common side effects of cholinesterase inhibitors include nausea, vomiting, and diarrhea. Weight loss can also occur. Deciding which of the three to use depends on patient and family preferences and tolerability (Qaseem 2008). All three come in pill forms and are taken on a daily basis. Rivastigmine is the only one that is also available in a patch form. It may be an alternative for someone with swallowing difficulties or a person who just prefers using a patch. However, it requires diligence in remembering when to take the patch off or put it on.

Donepezil is a popular choice to start with because of its simple regimen. It only needs to be taken once a day, compared to twice a day with galantamine and rivastigmine. Having to take a pill twice a day may not sound complicated, but if you have ever had to take antibiotics for a few days, you might recall those moments when you wonder whether you have taken your medicine for the day or not. Now, imagine having to take medicines twice a day for an extended period of time. This is in addition to the medications that one has to take for other medical issues. For someone with memory problems, having to remember to take a medicine once a day is much easier than trying to keep track twice a day.

When starting a cholinesterase inhibitor, as with taking many new medication, it should be introduced at the lowest starting dose. This is to ensure that the person does not experience an adverse reaction to it. Slowly increasing the amount of medicine to the optimal dose may allow the person to avoid side effects. For the most part, cholinesterase inhibitors are generally well tolerated. If someone develops side effects after taking a cholinesterase inhibitor, such as diarrhea, then the medication is usually stopped. Sometimes, the individual may find the side effect, such as nausea, tolerable, and wish to continue. Switching to another cholinesterase inhibitor is possible. However, because the medications have similar side effects, the individual can experience similar undesirable effects.

What happens if one agent does not appear to be effective? A discussion with the patient and family should be held about whether to continue treatment or consider another drug. Taking more than one cholinesterase inhibitor has not been studied and is not recommended. Sometimes loved ones enquire about stopping one cholinesterase inhibitor and trying another. Although the studies do not show one to be more efficacious than another, it may be worthwhile if the patient or family members are motivated to try. More frequently, depending on what stage of Alzheimer's disease the person is in, Namenda (memantine) may be added or substituted instead.

## MEMANTINE

Memantine acts differently from the cholinesterase inhibitors. The neurotransmitter regulated is glutamate. Glutamate is one of the principal neurotransmitters in neurons, in particular the neurons in the hippocampus, which is one of the main sites in the brain for storing memory. Once glutamate is released by a neuron, it carries information to other neurons, docking in receptors of the receiving neurons. One of those receptors is the N-methyl-D-aspartate (NMDA) receptor, which is involved in learning and memory. There is some data to suggest that insults, such as decreased oxygen from reduced blood flow in vascular disease, can lead to overstimulation of NMDA receptors. The NMDA receptors, when overstimulated, can be toxic to the neurons and lead to cell death. What memantine does is block glutamate from accessing the NDMA receptors, thereby preventing the receptors from being overexcited (Lancelot 1998). In this way, the neurons are protected from deterioration.

In 2003, memantine was approved by the FDA for use in individuals with Alzheimer's disease in the moderate to severe stages. Unlike cholinesterase inhibitors, which are recommended for use in early Alzheimer's disease, memantine is recommended for use in the more advanced stages. Many studies have shown memantine to be moderately effective in slowing the decline in mental capabilities (McShane 2006). These studies compare individuals with Alzheimer's disease who take memantine to others with the disease who do not take it. The drug's effect is measured by administering various memory and cognitive skills tests over a certain period of time. For example, the Mini Mental Status Exam (which we discussed in chapter 4) may be administered before starting memantine and again after a period of time to see if there is any significant change. These results are compared to individuals with Alzheimer's disease who are in a no-treatment group. Studies using different measures of memory and cognition have found that memantine can slow the decline a little bit as compared to the amount of decline in those who do not take it. However, how these improvements in test scores translate to real life is unclear. Nonetheless, memantine appears to have modest benefits in slowing deterioration in the moderate to severe stages of Alzheimer's disease.

Memantine is available in pill form. The recommended optimal dose is taken twice a day. As with cholinesterase inhibitors, it should be started at the lowest possible dose and slowly increased under the close supervision of a physician. The clinician may modify the dose depending on the individual's kidney function or tolerability. Memantine is generally well tolerated and found to have no significant adverse reactions compared to those people taking a placebo (a sham pill that does not contain actual medicinal properties) in some studies (Reisberg 2003). Dizziness appears to be one of the more common side effects. Rarely, hallucinations (or perceptions of images or sounds without an actual external stimulus) or worsening confusion can occur.

By the time someone is diagnosed with Alzheimer's disease, most are usually in the early to moderate stages. In these instances, starting treatment with a cholinesterase inhibitor is a reasonable choice. There is no recommended length of treatment. Usually, reassessment should be made after eight weeks of therapy to see how the individual is responding to the medication and whether there are associated undesirable effects. If there is some cognitive improvement, either by objective measurement or per family report, then the decision may be made to continue the drug. If there is no improvement, the decision to continue or discontinue therapy should be based on tolerability and patient and family preferences.

Sometimes after a period of treatment response, the individual may exhibit progressive cognitive decline as the disease advances. If the individual is already on the maximal dose of a cholinesterase inhibitor, memantine may be added. Some studies have shown treatment with a cholinesterase inhibitor in combination with memantine to have some benefit in behavior, cognition, and activities of daily living. Compared with individuals with moderate to advanced Alzheimer's disease who only take donepezil, persons who also take memantine appear to experience some benefit (Tariot 2004). Thus, for those people with more advanced Alzheimer's disease, adding memantine may be helpful.

## OTHER MEDICATIONS

Currently, cholinesterase inhibitors and memantine are the only drugs approved by the FDA for treatment of Alzheimer's disease. Researchers are working hard to develop better drugs that can potentially suspend or reverse the degeneration. Attempts to look at vitamins, estrogen (a female hormone that decreases after middle age), and herbs such as gingko biloba have been unsuccessful, and thus are not recommended. A type of pain medication called anti-inflammatory drugs (as the name suggests, these drugs work to decrease tissue inflammation) have also been studied, but in general have not shown any benefit in improving memory and cognition. There are numerous claims about the benefits of certain vitamins or herbs, but it is important to discuss them with a physician before starting any new medication.

## OTHER MANAGEMENT ISSUES

The management of Alzheimer's disease involves more than just treatment with medications. Caring for someone with Alzheimer's disease also necessitates addressing the various issues that arise as the dementia progresses. Some concerns that may arise are sleep disruption and weight loss. Behavioral disturbances also occur frequently. This usually requires non-pharmacologic interventions, that is, without using medications, although in some circumstances, medications may be necessary. Treating Alzheimer's disease also involves helping the individual maintain mental and physical function for as long as possible. Another important aspect is offering support to the caregivers, who are often family members. The responsibilities of providing care to someone with Alzheimer's disease can become burdensome. To care for a loved one day in and day out, for years on end, takes dedication and a lot of sacrifices.

## MANAGEMENT OF BEHAVIORAL SYMPTOMS

Behavioral disturbances, a broad term to describe changes in behavior that are out of the norm, are common manifestations of Alzheimer's disease. At times, managing the behavioral disturbances can be even more difficult for caregivers to cope with than the memory loss. Sometimes the behavioral disturbance is a change in personality or mood. Or it can be aggression or wandering. The individual may develop perceptual disturbances, called hallucinations. An attempt should always be made to handle disruptive behavioral symptoms non-pharmacologically first. However, in certain circumstances, medications may be necessary to keep the individual safe and comfortable. There is no easy solution to the various behavioral issues that may arise during the course of Alzheimer's disease. Sometimes a simple treatment is enough. Often times, multiple interventions are necessary, and even then it may not be enough to address the behavioral issues adequately. The well-being of the individual should always be the first and foremost consideration. Let's discuss some of the management issues that can arise as Alzheimer's disease progresses. However, please keep in mind that every person's symptoms and disease course will be different.

### Depression

*Mrs. Lee's children are worried about her. She stays in bed all day and sleeps most of the time. When they do convince her to join them for family activities, she complains of feeling tired and wants to go back to bed. She bursts into tears whenever her husband leaves her side. Her appetite has been poor. Even her grandchildren cannot cheer her up. They ask if this is a normal process of Alzheimer's disease.*

When depression occurs in individuals with Alzheimer's disease, it can be difficult to diagnosis. Recall that ruling out depression is necessary during the diagnostic process because depressive symptoms can mimic dementia. It is also known that elderly people with depression are at risk for developing cognitive impairment or dementia. So it is especially important that depression is recognized, diagnosed properly, and treated adequately.

Diagnosing depression in someone with Alzheimer's disease can be quite challenging. The individual may not have the self-awareness to recognize the symptoms. Or he may be unable to express himself clearly due to declining verbal abilities. For those people who are cognizant of the memory loss, being aware of their own progressive decline may bring about depressive symptoms. It may be especially true for those who are well educated or highly intelligent to have difficulty grappling with their worsening mental abilities. Furthermore, persons with Alzheimer's disease may develop mood changes such as sadness, apathy (lack of motivation), sleep problems, or decreased appetite due to the dementia process itself. This makes it tough to differentiate Alzheimer's symptoms from those of depression. Thus, diagnosing depression in Alzheimer's disease can be difficult.

Using traditional diagnostic tools to diagnose depression in someone with Alzheimer's disease may not be always feasible. Due to memory loss and language difficulties, the person may be unable to describe his mood and recent behavior. He may be reluctant to admit that anything is wrong. Or he may not even understand the questions being posed about his mood. Therefore, the diagnosis is usually based on descriptions provided by family members regarding any changes in behavior. Caregivers may describe crying spells, reluctance to participate in daily grooming, or decreased appetite. A gregarious individual may become one of sparse words. As alluded to before, the signs of Alzheimer's disease may not be easily distinguished from the symptoms of depression. In cases of uncertainty, it may be reasonable to treat the probable depression if there is a high index of suspicion.

Antidepressants (anti = against or in opposition) are medications used to treat depression. There are many antidepressants available, and some have been shown to be relatively well tolerated in the elderly. The clinician will select an antidepressant based on the individual's symptoms, while keeping in mind the potential side effects. Other health problems and medications are considered as well, in order to avoid any drug interactions or medical complications. As with starting any medication in a frail, elderly person with Alzheimer's disease, the chosen antidepressant should be started at the lowest dose possible and increased very slowly. Caregivers should be aware of the potential adverse effects so as to watch for them.

### Sleep

*Mrs. Lopez has been taking care of her husband with Alzheimer's disease for several years. Lately, she has been very tired from sleep deprivation. Her husband keeps her up almost every night with his antics. He wakes up an hour after going to bed and is up the rest of the night. He climbs up and down the stairs, goes to the bathroom hourly, and frequently rifles through this drawer or that closet. Not until the break of dawn does he fall asleep again. Mrs. Lopez does not know how much longer she can continue on like this.*

Sleep disruption can be common with the progression of Alzheimer's disease. As the disease process affects the brain center that controls sleep, the individual's sleep-wake cycle can become interrupted. Most of us structure our lives around our "internal clock," which allows us to maintain a normal sleep-wake cycle. This cycle usually consists of staying awake during the day and sleeping for a certain number of hours at night, but it can become disrupted in someone with Alzheimer's disease. Furthermore, even in healthy people, it is common for one to require less sleep as one grows older. As a result, a person with Alzheimer's disease may be up for part of the night or even all night in some cases. He may then sleep throughout the day. In extreme cases, the individual may stay up day and night.

The development of sleep disruption can be especially trying for family members who live in the same house. Imagine if you are woken up several times a night by the restless wandering of a grandparent throughout the house. Or by frequent toilet flushing. Or by the banging of activities within the house. Anyone would feel pretty tired and grumpy the next morning. Now imagine if this occurred every night and then you had to go to school or work the next day. This is not an uncommon scenario for many people who are caregivers to loved ones with Alzheimer's disease. Over time, it can be quite taxing physically and mentally to live with an Alzheimer's patient with disrupted sleep. It is nearly impossible to get restful sleep with the background noise. Out of safety concerns, a person with Alzheimer's disease should not be ignored if there is a risk of him wandering out of the house or taking a fall. Thus, not only is disrupted sleep concerning in an Alzheimer's patient, it also has a significant impact on the primary caregivers who share the same household.

The approach to managing sleep disturbance in Alzheimer's disease is dependent upon each individual's situation, with the goal of trying to regulate the person's sleep-wake cycle as much as possible. Efforts are made to identify those factors that may be contributing to the sleep disruption. Is the individual taking too many naps during the day? Drinking too much water after dinner, thus running to the bathroom in the middle of the night? Is he taking medications at night that are stimulating and preventing sleep? If this represents an acute change in behavior, a medical evaluation may be indicated to rule out underlying problems that may be contributing to the sleep disturbance.

When handling sleep disruption, caregivers are advised to keep the individual alert and engaged during the day. This may involve light exercises such as a daily walk or puttering around in the garden. The person is also encouraged to become engaged socially and mentally. One good way to achieve this is regular attendance of activities at the local senior center. Daytime naps are to be avoided if possible. Taking a nap in the afternoon can energize the individual so he or she will not be tired by bedtime. Napping can also cause disorientation; the person may wake up confused and thinking it is the next morning. Keeping the individual active during the day will help him sleep better at night (McCurry 2005).

In addition to daytime stimulation, it is important for individuals with Alzheimer's disease to keep as regular a routine as possible. This means keeping daily activities at the same time every day. Interrupting the schedule can lead to disrupted sleep. The person should try to wake up around the same time each morning, eat meals at set hours, and most importantly, go to bed at the same time at night. This may sound simple, but throw in a doctor's appointment or a visit by the grandchildren, the individual's routine can easily be thrown off track. Also, excessive stimulation, such as new visitors or activities, is discouraged in the evenings. Furthermore, maintaining the same routine before bedtime can be helpful. If the lights are dimmed and television turned off after a bath, the individual will come to associate these activities with sleep. Having the person go to the bathroom before getting into bed may avert the need to do it later in the night.

Another thing that caregivers can do to help their loved ones sleep better is to ensure their sleeping environment is comfortable. Is the person waking up because the room gets too cold in the wee hours of the night? Or is the comforter too thick and heavy, making it uncomfortably hot? Are the street lamps beaming too much light through the window? Adjusting the thermostat, changing the comforter and shutting the curtains are some examples of modifications that can be made to provide a pleasant environment. Furthermore, tripping hazards, such as electric cords or throw rugs, should be removed to prevent falls in case the person gets out of bed at night.

At times, despite the best efforts, the individual will still be unable to fall asleep or stay asleep. In situations like this, sleeping aids or medications with sleeping properties may be necessary. Sleeping medications that are readily available at the local drugstore should be avoided, as many have side effects that will do more harm than good. Any sleeping aid should be taken only under the supervision of a physician, as they may cause adverse reactions or interact with other medications. Plus, sleeping medications should only be administered after attempts at behavioral and lifestyle modifications are unsuccessful. They should be used in conjunction with continued behavioral interventions.

### Agitation and Aggression

*Mr. Bee calls his wife's doctor up in great distress. His wife, who has Alzheimer's disease, has become increasingly restless and confused in the afternoons for unclear reasons. She paces around the house and is unable to sit still. Several times, she has tried to leave the house, crying "I want to go home now!" When Mr. Bee attempts to stop her, she becomes even more upset and slaps him away.*

To become agitated is to be excited or upset emotionally. Many of us often take the ability to express ourselves for granted. To ask for food when we are hungry or seek help for a stomachache are acts we perform regularly without a second thought. But a person with Alzheimer's disease may be unable to express his needs or describe what is bothering him. Instead, agitation may be his way of expressing that something is wrong. The source of turmoil may be things that would not normally be upsetting, for example, a missing sweater. But for someone with dementia, he may not remember placing it in the laundry basket or make the connection to look in the dryer. Furthermore, the memory impairments often lead to confusion in new surroundings, or previously familiar things may appear strange and cause distress. Loss of verbal abilities can make it even more difficult for the person to describe his anguish.

For some people, the episodes of increased confusion and agitation predominantly occur later in the day. This phenomenon is called "sun-downing," as it occurs as the sun sets or in the late afternoon and can last into the night. Several explanations have been proposed for why this occurs, including fatigue and decreased lighting leading to shadows that are disconcerting.

In some situations, the person with Alzheimer's disease may exhibit aggression. Aggression is hostile behavior or attitude. In Mrs. Bee's case, she was slapping her husband. For others, aggression may present in the form of verbal barrages, such as cutting remarks or shouting profanities. In one instance, a former schoolteacher started cursing like a sailor at her daughter when she tried to administer her medications. Aggressive behavior can be very difficult for caregivers to handle.

Sometimes the agitation or aggression can be associated with delusions, which are false beliefs that are resistant to reason or evidence to the contrary. For example, the individual may accuse family members of stealing from him. It can be something as mundane as soaps or clothing, or as serious as money. Because the person is unable to remember where he left certain items, and even if he is shown where the missing item is located, he may not recognize the object or refuse to believe that it is the missing item. The delusions can also be of the paranoid type, where the person believes someone is coming after him. He may become suspicious of everyone around him. As you can imagine, these delusions can be quite distressing and, at times, even frightening. For someone with memory loss and trouble processing complex thoughts, he may not be able to understand when someone tries to reassure him that what he believes is false. In fact, he may get even more upset that no one believes him. He may become agitated, or react aggressively toward the caregiver, resulting in a vicious cycle.

In addition to delusions, a person with Alzheimer's disease may develop hallucinations as a result of the disease process, which can also be a great source of distress leading to agitation and even aggression. A hallucination is a sensory experience that feels real to the person, but does not exist outside of the mind. Visual hallucinations, or seeing objects that do not actually exist, can occur. Sometimes it can be small animals, such as dogs or cats, or humans. One elderly female would see her parents in the house, even though they died many years ago. Another person saw strange men in her bedroom. Auditory, or hearing, hallucinations can occur, but somewhat less frequently in Alzheimer's disease. Hearing voices or sounds that others do not can be frightening and easily cause agitation. As you can imagine, visual or auditory hallucinations can be quite scary to anyone. For someone with impaired mental abilities, the adverse effects of hallucinations can be exponential.

There are various potential explanations to consider when a person with Alzheimer's disease experiences agitation or aggression. Impairment of memory and cognitive ability can lead to confusion or misunderstanding, particularly if the individual cannot make himself understood. Delusions or hallucinations, especially frightening ones, can provoke agitation or restlessness. Depression can also result in altered behavior, as can chronic sleep deprivation. And multiple other issues, such as an acute medical illness, can also precipitate agitation. An individual with dementia may be unable to express himself if he is not feeling well; for example, if he has a toothache or a bladder infection. Thus, agitation or aggression in someone with Alzheimer's disease should not be simply taken for granted as a normal part of the disease.

When there is an acute change in behavior in an individual with Alzheimer's disease, he should be evaluated by a physician. The doctor will attempt to identify any precipitating cause. Family members should make note of and report any change in routine or environment. Sometimes a change in daily routine or the presence of a new face may be upsetting. Potential medical explanations are ruled out with a careful history, usually provided by the caregiver, and physical examination. A comprehensive review of the medications is necessary, in particular, examining any new medications. This is to ensure that the behavioral disturbance is not the result of adverse medication effects. Blood and urine tests may be performed to ensure there is no underlying medical abnormality, such as electrolyte imbalance or an infection. The physician may order more studies if necessary. If a potential cause is identified, then treatment is initiated to correct the problem, such as antibiotics for a bladder infection.

If there is no plausible medical explanation for the agitation, attempts should be made to manage the behavior without resorting to medications if possible. Because individuals with Alzheimer's disease get disoriented easily, avoiding new environments is recommended. For example, taking a parent with Alzheimer's disease to a relative's house for the holidays may seem harmless. Even though well-intentioned, it may prove to be too overwhelming and distressing, resulting in agitation. Being in an unfamiliar house, sleeping in a new bed, eating meals at different times and with relatives that he may no longer recognize—these can all lead to behavioral disturbances.

An unexpected change in daily routine can be upsetting to someone with Alzheimer's disease. It can cause disorientation, and should be avoided if possible. Another strategy is to avoid overstimulation, such as having too many visitors at once. For a person with memory loss, having numerous people come up to him can be overwhelming and lead to a change in behavior. When someone becomes agitated, it is also important to make sure the person's basic needs are met. Is he hungry? In pain? Tired? Soothing the person and keeping him comfortable can be helpful in calming him down. These are some strategies that can be applied, but it should be adapted to the situation on hand. For family members, it can be a lot like detective work trying to figure out what is bothering the loved one and what remedies will work.

A sole precipitating cause for the agitation may not always be readily identifiable. Usually, it may be a culmination of various factors. Sometimes treating what's believed to be the cause, such as an infection, may not improve the problematic behavior. When all possible causes have been explored, and there is no change in the agitation despite non-pharmacologic interventions, it may be necessary to use medications in some cases. When the behavioral disturbance can potentially bring harm to the individual himself or to the caregiver, such as in aggression, then using medications may help in some circumstances. Or they may help if the individual is having delusions or hallucinations that are quite distressing to him, such as seeing frightening men in his room or believing someone is coming after him. In such instances, using medications to treat these symptoms is reasonable.

When the symptoms of aggression, delusions, or hallucinations in Alzheimer's disease warrant treatment with drugs, a class of medications called antipsychotic drugs may be used. These medications are typically used to treat people with psychosis. Psychosis refers to mental disorders in which the person loses contact with reality and may have delusions or hallucinations. Antipsychotic ("against psychosis") drugs work to treat these symptoms of delusions or hallucinations. Although they are not approved by the FDA to treat behavioral symptoms in Alzheimer's disease, they are frequently used in clinical practice to manage behavioral disturbances that require pharmacologic treatment (Sink 2005).

Some studies have suggested that there may be a small increased risk of death associated with using certain types of antipsychotics in elderly people with dementia

(Schneider 2005). In fact, the FDA issued an advisory warning in 2005 requiring drugmakers to place this information on the labels (Food and Drug Administration). However, in special circumstances, such as if the delusions or hallucinations are causing significant distress to the Alzheimer's patient, the benefits of the medication may outweigh the risks. As with starting any medication, the family or caregiver should discuss the risks and benefits of the medication being proposed with the physician. Family members may be willing to accept the risks of side effects if the proposed antipsychotic drug is effective in providing relief from the behavioral disturbances. Currently, there are no medications available that specifically treat psychotic symptoms associated with Alzheimer's disease.

If the decision is made to treat with an antipsychotic drug, it should be started at the lowest dose and administered carefully. Deciding which antipsychotic drug to use typically involves consideration of the drug's side effects. As a class of drugs, antipsychotics have side effects that warrant cautious use. They can cause drowsiness, dizziness, and movement problems. They can worsen memory and confusion and they can also exacerbate certain preexisting medical conditions. Thus, antipsychotic drugs should be administered judiciously and under close supervision.

The newer, or second generation, antipsychotics are called atypical antipsychotics and tend to be favored over the older antipsychotics (also known as first generation or typical) for their side effect profile. The older, typical antipsychotics tend to cause more drowsiness, dizziness when changing positions, and heart problems. They are also more likely to result in movement problems such as tremors, muscle spasms, limb rigidity (or stiffness), and restless. The medical term for these types of movement disturbances is extrapyramidal symptoms. The extrapyramidal system in the brain controls motor movements. Sometimes, the person may appear as if he has Parkinson's disease, with hand tremors and slow, shuffling gait. Used long-term, typical antipsychotics can lead to a condition called tardive dyskinesia, which are muscle movements that a person cannot control, such as mouth twitching or arm flailing. Thus, atypical antipsychotics tend to be preferred over typical antipsychotics. However, because of the associated side effects with antipsychotic drugs in general, they should be used judiciously and under close supervision by a physician.

Besides antipsychotics, there are other types of drugs, such as mood stabilizers or anxiety medications, that may be tried, depending on the situation. The drug selected is dependent on numerous factors and more than one may be tried before an effective one is found. However, medications to treat behavioral symptoms in Alzheimer's disease should be of last resort and in conjunction with non-pharmacologic treatment strategies.

## Wandering

*Mr. Crown lives with his 80-year-old mother who has Alzheimer's disease. One day, while at work, his cell phone rang. It was the local hospital. His mother was in the emergency room. It turned out she was taken there by the police after being found wandering outside in her pajamas. She was almost run over by a car while crossing the street. Because she was unable to tell them where she lived or give the names of family members to call, she was taken to the hospital. Luckily, their neighbor happened to work there and recognized her.*

When wandering occurs in a person with Alzheimer's disease, it means that the person roams about unattended. Although the moving about may appear aimless to others, the affected individual may have a purpose or destination that may not be obvious. He may be searching for something, such as the bathroom or kitchen because he is unable to express urinary urge or hunger. Or the person may be looking for a familiar face. He may be disoriented and find his surroundings unrecognizable. It is not uncommon for the person to attempt leaving the house to "go home" or "go to work." He may be bothered by something in his current environment, such as a noise or shadow, and try to escape. Sometimes, there may be no clear explanation for the wandering. However, if a person has dementia, he is at risk for wandering (Rowe 2004).

Wandering can have very serious consequences in an individual with Alzheimer's disease. The person may be unable to find his way home. Or walk into oncoming traffic. Or fall and injure himself. The person may be lost for days without food or proper clothing. It is not unusual for an Alzheimer's patient found wandering to be taken to the hospital or police station because he is unable to recall his name or where he lives. When an individual starts wandering, it should be taken seriously. Steps need to be taken to ensure the person's safety.

As with onset of any behavioral disturbance, it necessitates a medical evaluation. It is important to rule out underlying medical conditions, such as an infection, that can worsen confusion leading to wandering. Medications should be reviewed to ensure it is not related to drug side effects. Caregivers should make note of any change in routine or environment that may have provoked the behavior change.

Wandering behavior creates a quandary for both the affected person and his loved ones. For those individuals living alone, this may signal the need for a more supervised living situation. If the person lives with family members, wandering can be difficult to handle. Family members may need to work and be unable to watch the person all day. There may not be the money available to hire someone to stay with the wandering individual. An elderly spouse who acts as the sole caregiver may be unable to keep up with a dementia patient who tries to leave the house. If wandering occurs at night, it can be even more arduous for caregivers to manage. Imagine how tiring it would be to stay up every night to prevent a loved one from leaving the house. Thus, the onset of wandering can be problematic in many respects.

What is a caregiver to do when the loved one starts to wander? It should be adapted to the individual's situation. It is important to ensure the person's basic needs are met, that he is not thirsty or hungry. Sometimes providing reassurance when the individual becomes anxious or disoriented can be helpful. If the person becomes restless, redirecting his attention to another activity may be efficacious. If there is no obvious reason for the wandering, one can consider providing a safe place for exploration, such as a path of certain rooms and hallways or a fenced backyard. If wandering out of the house is a major concern, one can try to camouflage the door by painting it the same color as the wall or covering it with a curtain. Child-proofing the doorknob is an option. Installing a bell may alert others when the door is opened. Some people have tried locking up or installing barriers to dangerous rooms, such as the stairway down to the basement. As every person's symptoms and living situation is different, the techniques for handling wandering should be tailored to the individual's needs.

Keeping the individual safe is of the utmost concern when there is a risk of wandering. There are some things that family members can do to protect their loved one from getting lost. Keeping an identification card or bracelet on the individual is one step. Sewing identification labels onto clothing is another option. The Alzheimer's Association has a Safe Return program designed to help return people who wander back to their families. With program enrollment, the loved one's information as well as emergency contacts are registered in a national database. In this way, if a person is found wandering, his family can be alerted. In addition to registering with a Safe Return program, it is also important to inform neighbors, the local police station, and nearby hospitals about the loved one's condition.

If the wandering behavior is frequent or persistent, it may no longer be safe for the person to be left unattended. However, it may not be feasible for caregivers to watch the person all day. Assistance from relatives or friends is sometimes available. Local elder service agencies may be able to provide a few hours of weekly care by a home aide. Some communities may have volunteer organizations that can provide companionship for a brief period of time.

However, the amount of care that these resources can provide is limited. Hired help for a certain time period, such as while the caregiver is at work, is available but not financially feasible for many people. In some instances, moving the person in with another family member who can bestow more care is possible. If there is no better alternative, transitioning the individual to a place where there is more supervision, such as a nursing facility, may be necessary.

## NUTRITION

*Mr. Grey has always enjoyed his food. He especially loves pastries—Danishes, croissants, muffins—he loves them all. However, lately, he no longer finishes his meals. Even when his wife places his favorite foods in front of him, he is uninterested in them. His wife has cut up his food into bite sizes and even tries to feed him to no avail. He refuses after a few bites.*

Weight loss and lack of nutrition are problems that can arise during the course of Alzheimer's disease. This can occur for many reasons. Early on, he may lose the skills to plan and prepare meals. He may forget how to use utensils. Later on, the person may lose appetite or motivation to eat. He may develop difficulty chewing food. He may need to be prompted to eat. In the advanced stages of Alzheimer's disease, swallowing difficulties arise. The food may go down the wrong way, called aspiration, and lead to lung infections. These are some of the issues surrounding nutrition and weight loss.

As the person with Alzheimer's disease develops increasing difficulty with eating, adjustments during meals can be tailored toward the person's needs. If the individual is having trouble using utensils, preparing foods that can eaten by hand makes it easier, such as sandwiches or fish sticks. Gently reminding the person to chew and swallow can help those who are pocketing food in their cheeks. Thickened liquids, such as pureed soups or shakes, can be tried if the person is coughing after swallowing thin liquids like water. There are also liquid thickeners available that can be added to any liquid. If chewing is the problem, soft foods that require less chewing can be attempted. Having the person sit upright during meals can help swallowing. Sometimes, an evaluation by a swallow therapist can teach the caregiver some techniques to promote eating.

Family members often have a hard time coping when their loved one is losing weight and having swallowing impairments. There is no easy solution. Because it is a common occurrence during the progression of Alzheimer's disease, there is no treatment to reverse the swallowing problem. In some medical illnesses, a temporary feeding tube may be an option to help the person receive nutrition until he is well enough to eat. One type of feeding tube is like a long, thin plastic straw that is inserted through the nose, down the throat to the esophagus and then the stomach.

Liquid nutrients are then plied into the tube. As the description implies, it is uncomfortable while it is inserted and while it is in place. Someone with Alzheimer's disease may not understand its purpose and pull it out. A more permanent feeding tube can be placed directly into the stomach by a minor surgical procedure. It is inserted through the abdominal wall directly into the stomach. Although a temporary feeding tube may be an option for certain medical conditions, is it helpful in Alzheimer's disease?

When eating becomes an issue in the advanced stages of Alzheimer's disease, the question of a feeding tube is often raised. It is difficult to witness a loved one lose weight. Family members worry about dehydration and hunger when their loved one stops eating. They worry about recurrent infections if the loved one is in and out of the hospital with aspiration pneumonias, or lung infections caused by food and secretions. However, studies have not shown feeding tubes to improve nutritional status in Alzheimer's patients nor have feeding tubes been demonstrated to prevent lung infections from aspiration. And the person does not live longer with a feeding tube. Thus, feeding tubes are not recommended for managing nutrition and weight loss in people with advanced Alzheimer's disease (Sampson 2009). However, this is a complicated issue that involves personal beliefs, cultural implications, and even religious convictions. Family members and caregivers should come to a decision that they are comfortable with after discussing the situation with their physician and considering all the facts.

## GAIT DISTURBANCE

*Mrs. Rice is brought into her doctor's office after a fall. Her daughter came home from work one day to find her lying on the kitchen floor. She had fallen and could not get herself up. Mrs. Rice could not say how long she was on the floor. Her daughter has been worried about her mother's ability to walk for a while. She is becoming progressively unsteady on her feet. She wobbles and holds onto furniture or leans on walls when she walks around her house. Her daughter is especially concerned about her climbing up and down the stairs.*

As Alzheimer's disease progresses, it is not uncommon for the gait, or the way a person walks, to become affected. The person will start exhibiting unsteadiness when walking. He may even fall, which can lead to serious injuries. Part of the management of Alzheimer's disease is encouraging the person to remain as physically active as possible. This is to maintain motor skills and preserve muscle strength. Caregivers are asked to encourage the person to perform physical activities on a regular basis. It can be activities that the person already enjoys, such as gardening or walking the dog.

When gait unsteadiness appears, physical therapy may be helpful. In addition to teaching exercises for leg strength and flexibility, the physical therapist can also identify problem areas in the gait and prescribe therapy as needed. Sometimes a gait assistive device may be necessary, such as a cane or walker, depending on the needs of the person.

## CAREGIVERS SUPPORT

Support for the caregivers is one of the most important aspects of managing Alzheimer's disease. Being a caregiver over a long period of time can cause stress and overwhelming burden, as well as adverse health effects. Thus, part of managing Alzheimer's disease is offering support to the caregivers while they deal with the various issues that arise throughout the disease course. This will be discussed in a later chapter.

The treatment strategy for Alzheimer's disease is a multipronged approach. Currently, there is no cure available. The available medications may slow the progression of the disease but do not reverse or halt the disease process. Thus, the treatment plan involves keeping the affected individual active physically, socially, and mentally, and maintaining function for as long as possible. It also involves supporting the caregiver over the course of the disease.

# 6

# The Course and Complications of Alzheimer's Disease

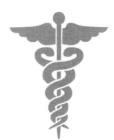

E ven though the term Alzheimer's disease was not coined until Dr. Alzheimer identified characteristic changes in Auguste D.'s brain in the early 1900s, this is not a new phenomenon that only came into being within the last century. The concept of dementia, or various forms of it, has been around for a long time. Deterioration of brain function with aging was described as early as 2000 B.C. by the ancient Egyptians (Boller 1998). It has also been mentioned in the writings of various Roman and Greek philosophers such as Plato and Hippocrates. Memory loss was once seen as a normal part of aging. But, as we have discussed, this isn't always the case.

The course of Alzheimer's disease is not the same for everybody. Some people live with it for a short period of time. Others may live with it for years, even more than a decade in some cases. Let's discuss the typical course of Alzheimer's disease, as well as some of the complications associated with it. Keep in mind that every person's symptoms and disease course will vary and may differ from what is described.

There are various frameworks used to describe the symptom patterns in Alzheimer's disease. These are usually in the form of classification systems, which attempt to group the symptoms into stages. Being able to describe Alzheimer's disease in stages is useful in helping patients and their families understand the disease better. It also assists them in anticipating future needs and planning accordingly. Some classifications may break it up into multiple numeric stages. Other frameworks simply divide it into a few stages, describing them in terms of disease severity—mild, moderate, and severe stages. However, even while using these classification systems, it is important to think of the disease process as a continuum, rather than distinct stages. There is no definitive line across which a person traverses into the next stage. Plus, it is not always easy to classify a person's symptoms into a particular stage, as they may overlap. Thus, while classification into stages is useful, one should also be mindful of the disease progression in a continuum.

## EARLY DISEASE

The changes of Alzheimer's disease often begin years before the affected individual shows any symptoms. In the earliest stages of Alzheimer's disease, there is no evidence of any impairment. The person does not exhibit any noticeable memory or cognitive problems. Family members do not suspect that anything is awry. Even to a physician, no obvious memory problems can be detected during routine checkups. While the degenerative process has begun in the brain, the disease burden has not reached the point of affecting the person's cognitive abilities noticeably.

Over time, the individual may become aware of his increasing forgetfulness. He may perceive brief memory lapses, such as forgetting where he placed his keys or glasses. The person may be a little slower to recall familiar faces or he may have occasional trouble remembering a certain word or phrase. However, this increased forgetfulness is not usually evident to close friends or family members. Evaluation by a health care professional may not reveal objective measurements of memory loss. The person may be reassured that what he is experiencing can be attributed to age-related changes. Nonetheless, a follow-up evaluation is indicated after a certain period of time to ensure there is no further decline.

## MILD DISEASE

After months to years have passed, the person's memory lapses may become more frequent and marked. The occasional missing keys may now be misplacement of valuable objects, such as a wedding band. He may have to read a newspaper article several times because he loses track of the story by the end. He may have difficulty with hobbies or duties he has performed for years, such as playing the piano or organizing family gatherings. Co-workers may remark on occasional lapses in performance. Family members may also start to notice increased absent-mindedness. Word-finding difficulties may start to show in conversations.

When the early changes of Alzheimer's disease become more noticeable, the person may initially be unfazed by them and simply attribute the problem to getting older. Close family members may also brush off the forgetfulness as an inevitable part of aging. The person may find it difficult to learn new information, such as the names of new acquaintances. He can have difficulty keeping track of recent events, such as what he did yesterday. He may forget important dates, such as a grandchild's birthday, or miss a dentist appointment. These may be simple annoyances at first, but as the occasional forgetfulness evolves into frequent occurrences, it becomes more difficult to ignore. This is usually when family members become worried to the point of seeking medical evaluation.

In the mild stage of Alzheimer's disease, the memory and cognitive deficits start affecting daily life. Short-term memory loss becomes more pronounced. The person may attempt to compensate by writing down things he needs to remember, such as transferring clothes from the washer to the dryer or paying the utility bills. However, he may start to repeat himself more as he is unable to remember what was just said. His children may notice that he will ask the same question repeatedly even though it has been answered, such as where they are going. Or he may ask what is for lunch when he ate it just an hour ago. These are some examples of pronounced short-term memory deficits that are apparent in the mild stage of Alzheimer's disease.

Another impairment that becomes evident in mild disease is difficulty with familiar tasks. A daughter became concerned when her mother could no longer operate the clothes washer, which is the same washing machine they have had for more than 10 years. She became even more worried when her mother stopped being able to manage her medications. Her mother was having trouble keeping track of which medications needed to be taken when. The person may forget the various steps involved in carrying out complex tasks that he used to perform without a second thought, such as balancing the checkbook or fixing appliances in his tool shed. He may also have difficulty with tasks that involve fine motor skills, such as dicing vegetables or typing on the computer. It may take him longer to complete these familiar tasks even though he used to perform them effortlessly. Mundane, everyday tasks can become increasingly hard for someone with Alzheimer's disease, especially as the disease progresses.

In addition to difficulty with routine tasks, learning new information and navigating unfamiliar environments becomes a challenge. Although we don't think about it consciously, we constantly encounter new people and surroundings as we go about our everyday lives. Even though we may take the same route to school or work every day, we walk by different people on the street and drive by different cars and objects daily, which can confuse someone with Alzheimer's disease. A person with Alzheimer's disease may have difficulty navigating in an unfamiliar environment. For example, a son noticed that when his elderly mother came to stay with him, she was a little disoriented and seemed lost in his house. As Alzheimer's disease progresses, the person will start to have difficulty even in a familiar environment. Objects may be misplaced not only due to forgetfulness but also due to decreased ability to recognize the objects.

Furthermore, the individual may also start having problems with everyday conversation. He may start to use the wrong terms in his conversations, such as saying tree when he means flower. Or if he has trouble recalling the name, he may try to describe it instead. Initially, the person may be able to circumvent the topic or compensate well in everyday conversation. However, his speech and language difficulties will become more noticeable as the dementia progresses.

Family members may also start to notice personality changes. A previously gregarious, outgoing person may become reserved and unwilling to go out anymore. The person may lose the motivation to golf or work on gardening projects like he used to. Co-workers may find him less motivated at his job. A previously easygoing person may become anxious and have temper outbursts. Sometimes, these personality changes may be more difficult for close family members to deal with than the memory loss.

Lack of insight may occur early on in Alzheimer's disease. A person who lacks insight has decreased abilities to see and acknowledge problems that he is having. He is unable to comprehend his deficits or he may underestimate the degree of the problem. In Alzheimer's disease, the affected individual may be unable to see his memory loss as abnormal. When family members start noticing and expressing concern about his memory, he may downplay the severity of it or the potential problems associated with it. Or he may not think he has memory loss at all. He may not believe he has cognitive impairments even when others try to explain them to him. Lack of insight becomes more pronounced as Alzheimer's disease progresses.

These are some examples of changes that may occur in mild Alzheimer's disease. The person may be exhibiting signs of Alzheimer's disease, but these changes usually have not yet affected the person's ability to function independently. The person may appear well but is actually having increasing difficulty with making sense of the world around him. Early on, he may be able to compensate for the cognitive changes and continue to function independently. However, as the impairments in memory and cognition become more marked, his daily functioning will become affected. Family members or caregivers may need to start providing assistance with activities of daily living, but the person may not rely on caregivers for everything. Spouses or children may take over managing the finances and administering medications. Caregivers may still feel comfortable leaving the person at home while they go out to work or for errands. Those individuals who live alone may still be able to do so with the supervision of caregivers checking in on them frequently.

## MODERATE DISEASE

As Alzheimer's disease advances, the symptoms become more pronounced and affect the individual's functioning more significantly. The memory loss becomes more obvious and more difficult to mask. The person will exhibit increasing signs of confusion, especially in unfamiliar environments or when subject to changes in routine. Even familiar surroundings may become difficult to navigate. Familiar objects may no longer be recognizable to the person. When the person starts having trouble recognizing friends and family members, it can be quite distressing for everyone. It is frustrating for the individual to not remember the name or recognize family members when it's expected of them. It is especially difficult and can be distressing for loved ones during these encounters. "Don't you remember me?" "You really don't know who I am?" These may be harmless questions, but they can exacerbate the frustration and confusion in a person with Alzheimer's disease.

Speech becomes more affected, and carrying on a conversation becomes more difficult. The individual will have trouble paying attention and following a conversation. He may repeat questions or statements over and over again. He may have more trouble expressing himself. His use of words and syntax may be jumbled. He may also have a hard time understanding others, such as instructions or explanations. This is often a point of contention and source of frustration for caregivers. Family members may try to explain something or give instructions, which the person may have difficulty understanding and following. Thus, both sides end up feeling frustrated. The affected person will have difficulty with complex thought processes and be unable to understand reasoning. For example, the person may start disliking bathing and resist attempts at grooming. He may become more upset at attempts to reason with him about the need for regular showers as he does not understand what is being asked of him.

He may have difficulty following favorite television shows due to shortened attention span and inability to understand the plot as well as being unable to commit it to short-term memory. He may forget the plot by the end of a show. Favorite activities such as reading may become difficult. This is due to a combination of various impairments, including inability to form short-term memory, language deficits, and decreased concentration. Writing is also affected. And working with numbers becomes a challenge. Not just complicated tax returns or a balancing checkbook but simple arithmetic such as counting out change or figuring out how many plates to set for dinner.

Difficulty with complex tasks becomes more prominent. The person with Alzheimer's disease will have trouble carrying out tasks that involve multiple steps. The tasks most of us perform on a regular basis without a second thought become difficult for someone with dementia. Examples include dressing, doing the laundry, and making a sandwich. Something seemingly simple, such as making a cup of tea, actually requires multiple steps, which becomes progressively difficult for someone with cognitive impairment. Imagine the steps, which include filling the kettle, turning on the stove, waiting for the water to boil, putting a teabag into a mug. Once the kettle whistles, turn the stove off, and pour water into the mug without burning one's hand on the hot kettle. These various steps require concentration, remembering the necessary sequence, and motor coordination, all of which are skills impaired in Alzheimer's disease.

Problems with executive function also become more pronounced in the moderate stages of Alzheimer's disease. Not only does the person have problems with carrying out familiar tasks, he also has trouble with planning and executing new tasks. Due to difficulty organizing his thoughts and thinking logically, the individual will find it hard to plan and carry out various activities. Preparing a meal requires mentally planning out the recipe and necessary ingredients. Leaving the house to go to a hairdresser's appointment also necessitates advanced planning. Furthermore, the person may be unable to cope with new or unexpected situations. Whereas he used to find it difficult, he may no longer be able to adjust or react to new or unpredictable environments.

In moderately advanced Alzheimer's disease, behavioral changes occur more frequently. Some examples include restlessness and agitation. He may become tearful and increasingly confused toward the end of the day, also known as sun-downing. The person may develop hallucinations, such as seeing dead family members, or it may involve animals or strangers in his room, which can cause significant distress. He may also develop delusions. He may accuse family members of stealing from him, despite being shown the missing item. Or he may be frightened that someone is coming after him. He may become suspicious of everyone around him. He may become irritable and have anger outbursts out of proportion to the situation or without clear reason. Or rather, the person may become increasingly anxious about everything, such as when his wife or caregiver is out of sight. On the other hand, the person may become withdrawn and unmotivated.

Another behavioral change that can occur is loss of impulse control. As we are growing up, we are taught to behave in particular ways in public, such as dressing appropriately and using acceptable language. We learn to control our impulses if they are inappropriate, such as not laughing at a funeral or interrupting someone in the middle of her speech. As Alzheimer's disease progresses, this ability is lost. The person may leave the house in her nightgown or even start to undress in public. Or she may try to hug strangers and not find it inappropriate.

As Alzheimer's disease progresses from mild to moderately severe stages, the various symptoms of memory loss and cognitive deficits become more pronounced. The individual also exhibits pronounced problems with speech and language, as well as learned motor skills. His gait, or ability to walk, will progressively become slower and more unsteady. He may need a cane or walker but will often forget either when he wants to walk somewhere. Falls and injuries from falls may occur. His sleep-wake cycle may become disrupted.

Most concerning is when these changes affect the individual's ability to carry out his daily functioning. Family members or caregivers who are involved may try to assist the person to the best of their abilities. They may cook or bring food, manage the finances, and fill medication prescriptions. They may assist with grooming or bathing as needed. However, this may not be enough as the Alzheimer's disease worsens. If the individual lives alone, his memory and cognitive impairments will eventually reach the point when it is not feasible for him to live alone. Even if the person lives with a spouse or other family members, his impairments may worsen to the point where they can't be managed. This may occur when behaviors such as wandering or aggression become too much for family members to handle.

Whether he lives alone or is home alone during the day while family members work, if the person starts exhibiting wandering, then it may be unsafe for that individual to remain home alone. It may be necessary to hire a companion, which can be costly depending on the amount of time needed. In some cities, there are senior or elderly centers that provide day care services. If this is available, it is often encouraged as it gives the person structured social stimulation as well as physical activity. It also allows caregivers a much-needed break from their duties. This is also an option if the individual lives alone. However, there may come a point when it is no longer feasible for the person to live alone or at home. There are facilities available called assisted living or dementia units, which will be discussed in a later chapter.

Another issue that arises is driving, or rather, when to stop driving. This is often a sensitive topic to raise with someone with Alzheimer's disease. Obtaining a driver's license for the first time as a teenager is frequently equated with a newfound freedom. Thus, to take away someone's driving privileges is to remove someone's independence. Especially for someone who has been driving for decades, it can be quite devastating. Frequently, even though the person has obvious difficulties with driving, he lacks insight and cannot recognize the problems or potential danger in continuing to drive. There is no clear-cut answer to when exactly a person should stop driving. If the person is getting lost or into mishaps while driving early on, then he should stop driving even if a diagnosis of Alzheimer's disease has not been made. Once diagnosed, the person himself and even family members may feel comfortable allowing him to continue to drive for the time being. However, it may be necessary to administer a driving evaluation to assess the person's driving capabilities, and a discussion should be initiated early on about planning for when it is no longer safe for the person to drive. Alternative modes of transportation should be looked into. Sometimes it may be necessary to take away the car keys against loud protest by the affected individual. Some states require a physician to report if a patient's medical condition precludes him or her from driving. This is an issue that should be addressed early on, and ultimately, the person will lose the ability to drive.

## SEVERE DISEASE

As Alzheimer's disease progresses into the end stages, the individual continues to decline mentally and physically. The memory loss deteriorates to the point where he no longer recognizes anybody, not even his closest loved one. All aspects of bodily function are significantly impaired as the disease ravages every corner of the brain. From his use of arms and legs, gait, speech, and swallowing to control of bladder and bowel function—no function is left untouched in the final stages of Alzheimer's disease.

The individual's gait will continue to deteriorate, from needing a cane to a walker, to needing assistance to get up from a chair or out of bed. His legs will get weaker and weaker, and walking more unsteady, needing to be propped up as he walks. The deterioration continues until the person will stop walking all together. He will need someone to pick him up out of bed and transfer him to a wheelchair or chair and vice versa. Even sitting up may not be feasible. In addition to the loss of use of the legs, all motor functions deteriorate and become impaired. The initial struggles with using his fingers, in activities such as buttoning or eating, deteriorate until the person stops using his arms purposely. He will stop being able to do things such as putting on clothes, brushing his teeth, or feeding himself. He will need someone to help him with all these activities that he is no longer able to do for himself.

The memory loss deteriorates to the point where the person has little memory left, neither short-term nor long-term. He will no longer be able to recognize his closest family members. Calling his name may be met with a blank look. His language and speech will continue to decline. He may repeat phrases that do not make sense or be unable to answer questions appropriately. Or he will call out names or phrases repeatedly, without knowing what he is really asking for. He will say less and less, until he barely speaks at all.

Weight loss is a common complication at the advanced stages of Alzheimer's disease. The person will develop difficulties with eating. He will lose the initiative to eat and need to be prompted to put food in his mouth. He will also forget what to do with the food once it's in his mouth. It is not uncommon to find bits from the previous meal sitting in his cheek pockets. He needs to be reminded to swallow, which is another problem that arises. Like all motor functions, swallowing is a complex process controlled by the brain and carried out by the muscles in the mouth and throat to move food from the throat into the esophagus, or passageway into the stomach. The trachea, or airway passage into the lungs, sits right in front of the esophagus. With breakdown of the swallowing mechanism, food or liquids can go down the wrong passageway and end up in the lungs. It can even occur with swallowing saliva. In medical terms, this is called aspiration. And it can lead to aspiration pneumonia, which is lung infection caused by aspiration.

It causes great distress to family members to see their loved one stop eating. The person loses weight and becomes frail. The urge will be to find ways to encourage the individual to eat more. When regular solid foods are no longer feasible, soft or pureed foods are recommended. Thicker liquids, such as milkshakes, are preferred over thin liquids, such as water, as thicker liquids are less likely to cause choking or aspiration. Caregivers are encouraged to hand-feed the food, as it also increases the amount of face to face interaction with the person. Feeding tubes are not recommended for people with advanced Alzheimer's disease. They do not prevent aspiration pneumonias or improve nutritional status or weight gain.

Incontinence, or loss of bladder or bowel control, is another inevitable part of advanced Alzheimer's disease. The person may develop urinary incontinence in the earlier stages of dementia, where he may occasionally leak when he is unable to make it in time. It continues to worsen until he stops getting the urge to go the bathroom and is unable to ask for assistance when he feels the urge. The same is true for bowel movements. Adult diapers are frequently used. Thus, caregivers are very important as the person with advanced Alzheimer's disease relies on his caregivers to change the diapers. It is important to maintain cleanliness to avoid skin breakdown and infections around the area.

This brings us to another complication of end-stage Alzheimer's disease, which is skin ulcer. A skin ulcer is an open sore in the skin that often looks like a crater. Remaining in one position for too long can lead to skin breakdown, especially in those areas with extra pressure, such as the buttock, heels, and elbows. As the individual becomes bed bound, he will frequently lay in one position for prolonged periods until someone turns him. Sitting in a wheelchair for an extended period of time poses the same risks. Even with changing positions, the trauma on the skin from shifting him in bed, such as turning him to change sheets or clothing, can lead to skin break down. Poor nutritional status places the person at risk for skin breakdown and also comprises wound healing. The ulcer may be shallow at first and worsen to the point where bone is visible. Wound care is particularly important to prevent worsening of the ulcer, as well as to prevent infections. In particular, ulcers that develop on the buttock are more susceptible due to potential exposure to urine and feces. A fatal complication may result from an ulcer infection that invades the bloodstream and causes a systemic infection.

By the time someone reaches the severe stages of Alzheimer's disease, he will require total care. Some caregivers may choose to take care of the individual around the lock, but this is not always an option. It is a demanding role that is taxing mentally, physically, emotionally, and financially. Some families may take shifts taking care of the person. Others may be able to hire personal care attendants to help with the caregiving tasks. However, placement in a nursing home may be necessary if the person is unable to receive the necessary care at home. It is a difficult and often heart-wrenching decision for anybody to make, but sometimes, it may be the only option. Discussion and planning for what to do in the advanced stages of Alzheimer's disease should be initiated early on.

At the end stage of Alzheimer's disease, the person will have deteriorated to a shadow of his former self. He will be bedridden, nonverbal, and barely interactive with those around him. He is often emaciated and incontinent. He will be dependent on those around him for his basic needs. Persons with Alzheimer's disease frequently die of complications from the disease, such as infections. Pneumonia and urinary tract infections are common infections that occur. Serious infections from skin ulcers can also complicate the process. Other causes of death may be medical issues such as a heart attack or stroke.

The various stages and progression of Alzheimer's disease occur over a period of years. What is described above is a typical course. However, every person's symptoms and complications are different. After a diagnosis of Alzheimer's disease is made, the individual and family members should become educated about the course of Alzheimer's disease so that potential problems and complications can be anticipated. It is a bleak picture. The goal is to help the person remain comfortable and dignified as he goes through this process.

# 7

# How Does Alzheimer's Disease Affect the Family and Caregivers?

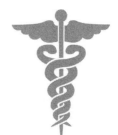

*An anxious Mrs. White comes into her doctor's office complaining of an abnormal spot on her skin. Despite her doctor's reassurance that it is nothing worrisome, she continues to be worried that it is cancerous. She becomes tearful as she describes her daily life taking care of her husband with Alzheimer's disease for the last five years. She frequently worries about what would happen to him if something happened to her. There is no one else to take care of him.*

Alzheimer's disease not only affects the patient but also the people around him. The lives of family members, especially those directly involved in the individual's care, are significantly impacted in many ways. For the primary caregiver involved in the day-to-day care, the disease can take a toll emotionally, physically, mentally, and financially. The responsibilities of a caregiver may extend many years, depending on the course of Alzheimer's disease in the loved one. Not only does the caregiver have to witness the progressive deterioration in her loved one, she also has to cope with the various symptoms and complications that can arise. Let's discuss the impact of Alzheimer's disease on family members and caregivers. We will also review some advices and resources to help caregivers in handling their responsibilities.

## IMPACT ON THE FAMILY

Even before a diagnosis is made, close family members will have witnessed the memory decline and suspect something is not quite right. However, having their suspicions confirmed does not make it any easier to come to terms with the diagnosis. It can be a devastating diagnosis to receive, especially for those people who have witnessed the decline of, or even cared for, someone with Alzheimer's disease. Coming to terms with having a close family member diagnosed with Alzheimer's disease can be difficult. There may be misconceptions about the disease, such as that it is nothing more than memory loss. The fact that it is a progressive, and ultimately terminal, illness can be difficult to grasp. The diagnosis of a parent or spouse with Alzheimer's disease may also conjure up a number of mixed emotions, such as frustration, helplessness, or even guilt. As every person handles his emotions differently, addressing the various feelings is an important part of coming to terms with the diagnosis.

Just as the affected individual's life is altered inexorably, so are the lives of his caregivers in many aspects. One of the major changes is a change in roles. A son or daughter may be used to playing the role of the child, sometimes well into adulthood. A child accustomed to having her parents dote on her may suddenly find herself in the role of the caregiver. This reversal of roles from being the child to the nurturing care provider can be unsettling and even overwhelming. It can be quite difficult to witness a previously vibrant and independent parent decline over time to a former shadow of himself. Having to adjust to increasing responsibilities as a caregiver can be taxing emotionally and psychologically. This role reversal also occurs frequently for spouses. A husband whose wife has always managed the household may find himself having to take over, or vice versa. It is not uncommon for a husband used to having his wife take care of his daily needs to struggle with learning to meet her needs. Grandchildren may find themselves having to take over as the caregivers. Sometimes, a niece or nephew will find themselves in the role of caregiver. Whatever the makeup of the family, there is usually a change of roles, and someone steps into the shoes of caregiver.

### Health Impact

As Alzheimer's disease progresses, the individual's needs increase too, resulting in increased demands on the caregiver. Whether the caregiver lives with the affected individual or not, the responsibilities of a caregiver can have significant impact on one's life. Over time, the burden of caregiving can lead to medical problems, such as depression and anxiety. The stress of caring for a person with Alzheimer's disease can also take a toll emotionally and physically. And it can affect the caregiver's overall health as his own health issues may be neglected due to the demands of caregiving. Thus, the burden of caring for someone with Alzheimer's disease can have a negative effect on the caregiver's health.

In the early stages of Alzheimer's disease, the demands on the caregiver may not be too demanding. It may be enough for the caregiver to check in on the parent or grandparent once a day. Or the caregiver may still be able to leave the house to go to work or run errands. This allows the caregiver to maintain some semblance of her daily routine without too much disruption. However, as the affected individual's memory and cognition deteriorates further, he will need more assistance with daily activities. The person may become upset when his wife attempts to leaves the house. He may start wandering out of the house. Or he may fall frequently while home alone. It may reach the point where it is no longer safe for the person to be left home alone for extended periods of time. These are some of the issues that the caregiver has to face, and, sometimes there are no easy answers.

As the affected individual increasingly relies on his spouse or child, it poses a greater burden on the loved one providing care. It may lead to caregiver burden, which is a term used to describe the physical, emotional, and financial toll of providing care. Some caregivers may feel the strain in one particular aspect, whereas many experience the toll across the whole spectrum. Studies have shown that family caregivers are more likely to experience symptoms of depression and anxiety compared to people who are not caregivers (Cochrane 1997). Spouses who care for a husband or wife with a chronic illness are much more at risk for depression and anxiety compared to children caring for a parent. Depression and anxiety are medical conditions that have an impact on overall health and need to be treated. Furthermore, studies have found elderly people who have their own chronic illnesses and are experiencing caregiving-related stress have a much higher rate of death than caregivers who do not experience stress (Schulz 2001). Caring for people with dementia can also impact a person's immune system and lead to an increased chance of developing medical illnesses. Thus, the strain of caring for someone with Alzheimer's disease can have significant impact on one's health.

### Financial Impact

Caring for a loved one with Alzheimer's disease can become a burden financially. Many people are unprepared for the expense of caring for someone with dementia. The costs can be indirect, such as loss of work time or expenses for traveling back and forth to care for the person. It is not uncommon for a caregiver to use up all her sick and vacation days to provide care. Sometimes, jobs may be placed in jeopardy due to the demands of caregiving.

The total tab of direct care can add up exponentially as the needs of the person increase. It can include doctors' office visits and medications. Equipment may be necessary, such as walkers or home alterations to make the home safer. Health care supplies, such as diapers or dressings, can be expensive. Perhaps one of the more costly expenses is hired companions or home aides. Depending on the number of hours and the types of services needed, the cost of hiring someone to take care of a loved one with Alzheimer's disease can be quite costly. If the caregiver is unable to care for the affected individual at home, then the cost of a skilled nursing facility is another expense to deal with.

The expense of caring for someone with Alzheimer's disease can be unexpected, and, for many people, become a burden. This may be especially true for a retired, elderly couple on a fixed income, as well as for people with their own families and health issues to take care of. Managing the financial burden of the care can pose significant stress on a caregiver.

### Emotional Impact

In addition to the health and financial burdens that caring for someone with Alzheimer's disease pose, it also takes a toll on the caregiver emotionally. Caring for someone around the clock, day in and day out, for months or years on end can have significant impact on a person emotionally. In dealing with the various behavioral issues that arise, it is only human to react accordingly. For example, feeling frustration at spilled milk or feeling hurt at a cutting remark. Even while understanding that the words and behaviors are unintentional and due to the disease process, having to restrain typical emotions can be trying. Plus, not being appreciated by the loved one for the sacrifices the caregiver is making can make it less rewarding.

Furthermore, providing care can be like an emotional roller coaster. One may experience the whole spectrum of feeling over the course of a day as a caregiver. These include frustration when the person does not follow directions despite repeated attempts or anger at the person for soiling his pants, and then feeling guilty afterward for raising one's voice to laughing at a comical moment. Then, the next minute, feeling sad and hurt at being accused of stealing. These are some examples of the emotional turmoil that can occur as a caregiver, which can be compounded by health issues, fatigue, and financial worries. If not dealt with properly, these strains can lead to more serious mood problems such as depression.

### Physical Impact

The physical burden of caring for a person with Alzheimer's disease can become overwhelming. As the individual's cognition deteriorates, it becomes necessary for someone to always be present to prevent harm and ensure basic needs are met. This can be quite demanding on the caregiver physically.

As the affected individual becomes weaker physically, he becomes increasingly reliant on his caregiver. He may require assistance with getting in and out of a chair, or in and out of a tub. For a wife trying to help her husband who outweighs her by 100 pounds, this may be near impossible. The caregiver may need to wake up several times a night to assist with bathroom trips or to ensure safety if the person he is caring for is wandering or not sleeping. Alzheimer's patients with a disrupted sleep-wake cycle who are up most of the night can keep the entire household up with him. The chronic lack of, or continually disrupted, sleep can be immensely taxing on the caregiver and affect overall health. It can cause irritability and emotional ups and downs. If the caregiver has no one to help relieve him and allow time to rest and decompress, the fatigue can be compounded.

## COPING AS A CAREGIVER

Frequently, people are thrown into the role of the caregiver for their loved one with Alzheimer's disease without being prepared. It is usually an unexpected position that one is placed in. As there is no school or course for this, caregivers find themselves learning as they go along. Caregivers often need to juggle their own lives while trying to take care of the loved one with Alzheimer's disease. Over time, the responsibilities as a caregiver can impose significant strain and stress, and even lead to caregiver burden. Let's discuss some ways to help a caregiver cope with the burdens that accompany the responsibilities.

### Recognize the Warning Signs

The strain of caring for someone with Alzheimer's disease puts one at increased risks for problems such as depression and anxiety. Furthermore, the responsibilities may lead the caregiver to neglect his own health, which can lead to serious medical issues. Thus, it is important to recognize the warning signs of caregiver burden and seek help before it becomes more serious. It is also critical to acknowledge depressive symptoms or signs of deteriorating health to avoid adverse complications. These problems may also affect the ability to provide care.

Sometimes, the strain of providing care can lead to inadvertently taking out the frustration on the person being cared for, which is a serious matter. Thus, recognizing the warning signs of caregiver burden in a timely manner is important.

What are some of the warning signs to be aware of? If the caregiver is experiencing emotional problems, poor sleep, decreased appetite, sadness, crying spells, these can be symptoms of depression. These symptoms may be signs of other mood disorders or herald other medical illnesses. Sometimes, the caregiver may be unaware that these symptoms are out of the norm or concerning. They may be brushed off or minimized as he or she is so focused on caring for the loved one. However, it is important for the caregiver to recognize the warning signs, or acknowledge them if those around him are expressing concern. It is important to seek timely medical evaluation to receive a proper diagnosis and treatment.

### Finding Time for Rest

One of the most important things to do as a full-time caregiver for someone with Alzheimer's disease is to find time for rest. Although it may sound like common sense, it is more difficult than it sounds. The person absorbed in caring for a loved one with Alzheimer's disease may not recognize the need for rest and relaxation. He or she may even feel guilty about spending time away or doing something enjoyable without the loved one. Or there may be no one available to relief the caregiver.

However, finding time to rest does not necessarily mean going out to have fun. It means that the caregiver must be allowed adequate time for rest, whether it is a half an hour a day to just sit down or finding the time to catch up on sleep. It may also mean making sure the caregiver allows herself to sit down to enjoy her meals, rather than eating standing or jumping up frequently to attend to the loved one. These are just some examples of things that a caregiver can do to give herself a break. Finding time for rest should be an integral part of caregiving. Whether it be an hour to herself while the loved one is taking a nap, or allowing other family members or friends to take over for an afternoon. It is important for the mind, body, and soul. Otherwise, the burdens of providing care may become too overwhelming and have an adverse impact on the caregiver.

Finding the time to attend to one's health is also an integral part of caregiving in order to avoid the consequences of stress and burden. This means making time to see one's physician regularly for checkups. When doctor's appointments collide, it is not uncommon for a caregiver to cancel her own in order to ensure her husband does not miss his appointments. Thus, making time for one's own appointments is important, whether it be with a dentist or for an eye exam. It is important to not just brush off any signs of illness in favor of caregiving duties. It is also important to manage one's medications properly, to take them on time and as prescribed. Some caregivers may monitor the loved one's health status carefully but forget that he needs to manage his own medical issues as well, such as monitoring blood sugars or blood pressure. Thus, ensuring that time is set aside to attend to personal needs is a crucial part of coping as a caregiver. Allowing one time to rest and recharge not only maintains overall health, it is important to carrying out the responsibilities of caring for someone.

### Support Groups

In addition to finding protected time to rest and attend to personal needs, it is also important to find an outlet to express one's frustrations as well as sharing feelings about caring for someone with Alzheimer's disease. Being the primary caretaker for someone with this disease can be isolating, as most of one's time is consumed with caring for that person. Plus, other family members or friends who are not directly involved may not understand the emotional and psychological stress involved. And even though friends and family may be supportive, it might not be enough. Thus, it is helpful and often therapeutic to share one's experience with other people who are going through a similar experience.

There are various support groups available for people who care for a loved one with Alzheimer's disease. The types of support groups available depend on the community in which one lives. There may be a group just for wives caring for husbands or vice versa, or children caring for a parent. Being able to meet others in the same situation and sharing experiences can relieve stress and also validate one's role as a caregiver. Valuable tips on managing the various issues that come up in caring for a dementia patient can be gleaned as well. Sometimes, friendships may be formed, and giving each other support over the phone can be invaluable. Local elder service agencies or Alzheimer's groups may also have hotlines for caregivers to call for advice. Another forum to meet people in similar situations is online support groups. For caregivers who are shy or unable to leave the home, joining an online support group or chat room may be helpful as well.

Sometimes speaking with strangers at a support group may not be appealing. In these situations, regular sessions with a therapist may be helpful. Therapists are trained to help an individual work through his or her internal turmoil. Thus, discussing one's emotions with a therapist may help alleviate some of the strains one experiences from caring for someone with Alzheimer's disease. Another benefit of seeing a therapist is the confidentiality factor, as some people may feel uncomfortable in sharing with others who also live in the same community.

### Respite Care

Sometimes, the burdens of caring for someone with Alzheimer's disease can be quite overwhelming. For those people who dedicate themselves entirely to providing care, the stress of caregiving over time can take a significant toll on a person mentally, emotionally, and physically. Some people may be the sole caregiver without any outside help. Respite care should be considered when the caregivers burden becomes too much. It is important as a regular part of caregiving so as to allow the caregiver time to rest and take care of himself. Respite care is short-term or temporary relief to those people who provide long-term care for someone with a serious illness. It gives the caregiver a break from the monotony and strain of daily tasks that leave little time for rest.

Respite may be a few hours a day or a week provided by family, friends, hired companions, or even volunteers. Or it may be for a few days or weeks. There are various settings for respite care. As mentioned, relatives or friends may be able to stay over to allow the caregiver some time off. Some elderly service agencies or community organizations such as the local Alzheimer's association may be able to provide volunteers or companions at a reduced rate. Another type of respite care for a few hours is adult day care. Some senior centers may provide adult day care where the loved one can go for several hours during the day, as frequently as several days a week, to allow the caregiver some respite.

For respite care of longer duration, such as several days or weeks, some cities have specialized housing or nursing homes where people with significant nursing requirements may stay temporarily. These facilities may be available for emergency situations as well, for example, if the caregiver has an urgent medical issue.

## RESOURCES AND SUPPORT FOR THE CAREGIVER

### Becoming Educated

One of the most important things for family members to do once their loved one is diagnosed with Alzheimer's disease is to become educated about the disease. Learning about it will help the caregiver cope better as the disease progresses. It also allows the caregiver to anticipate problems that may arise. Understanding the disease process and potential complications empowers the caregiver to feel prepared and less helpless. Learning about the disease may also help the caregiver regain some sense of control over the situation and aid in alleviating the feeling of helplessness.

There are various resources available to learn about Alzheimer's disease. The physician is a good place to start. It is helpful to write down questions before regular office visits. The doctor will usually be able to provide pamphlets or make suggestions about available resources. A lot of people turn to the Internet for medical information these days. There are some reputable sites that are informative (refer to list at the back). However, not all sites are fact-checked or have reliable sources, and some may provide incorrect information or promise treatments that are not validated. Thus, it is important to be cautious when gleaning information from the Internet and use those sites that are reputable or affiliated with a trustworthy organization.

The library or bookstore is also a good place to learn more about Alzheimer's disease. Many books have been published on this topic, and some are tailored toward caregivers. In addition, the local Alzheimer's organization can be an invaluable resource. They frequently put out publications and even regular newsletter to keep interested people up-to-date. These are some examples of resources available for caregivers to better understand Alzheimer's disease and in turn, help them cope better and provide better care.

### Planning for the Future

Once a loved one is diagnosed with Alzheimer's disease, it is important for the family members to start planning for the future. Depending on what stage of disease she is in, the person may live with it for many years. For the family, this means that their responsibilities as caregivers may last for a very long time. Caring for someone with Alzheimer's can be quite costly, and family members should plan early on for how to meet the expenses. It may involve meeting with an accountant or financial advisor to better understand the available options. It is also important to learn about health insurance and the potential costs of health care in various settings, as it can be quite complicated. Becoming educated as soon as possible about what resources are available to help defray some of the costs can be helpful later on.

The affected individual and her family members should also meet with a lawyer in a timely manner. This is to discuss paperwork in preparation for the time to come when the loved one with Alzheimer's is no longer able to manage her own finances or other legal matters. Depending on the state laws, separate legal paperwork may be put in place stating the person's wishes for medical treatments as well as appointing someone to be her representative in making health decisions. These are important issues that should be discussed and put in place early on.

In addition to planning financially and legally, it is also important to plan for future settings of care. If a wife is the primary caregiver, what happens to her husband if she becomes ill or passes away? If a person with Alzheimer's disease lives alone and has no relatives or friends, someone from the local elder services agency may need to become involved and help plan for future care. Or if it is no longer feasible for the person with Alzheimer's disease to live at home, alternative arrangements should be found, such as an assisted living facility or even a nursing home. These are some common scenarios that arise. Even though not every person's situation is the same, it is important for the planning to begin early on.

### Case Manager

A geriatric case manager can be invaluable to caregivers of persons with Alzheimer's disease. A case manager can guide the person in navigating the various aspects of the health care system, especially with regard to the different levels and types of care. Geriatric case managers are specialized in helping elderly persons and their families navigate the health care system with special attention to the needs of the elderly. The health care system is a huge labyrinth of different facilities, from hospitals to nursing homes, that provide different levels of care. It can be confusing for a caregiver to figure out what is the best type of care or care setting as the loved one progresses through the various stages of Alzheimer's disease. For example, a daughter trying to find a safer living environment for her mother may be uncertain about the difference between an assisted living facility and nursing home. A case manager can help relieve some of the stress and burden by assisting in this process.

### Social Worker

Having a social worker can help caregivers in many ways. A social worker helps individuals function in their environments and manage their relationships, and assists in dealing with personal and family problems. Geriatric social workers are trained to assess the social needs of the elderly person. They often act as the link between the elderly person and community agencies and services. This can be particularly valuable to persons with Alzheimer's disease and their families. The social worker can help them access services or programs that they may otherwise not know about, such as home health aides or special transportation. Some social workers also have extra training in mental health and can provide therapy for persons with depression or anxiety. Thus, social workers can be a good resource for caregivers. They are readily accessible through various settings, such as hospitals or the local elder services agency.

### Accepting Help

For some caregivers, asking for or accepting help does not come easy. There are many devoted husbands and wives who dedicate themselves completely to their responsibility in taking care of their spouse with Alzheimer's disease. This is also true for many children or grandchildren caring for their elder relatives. Sometimes, they may feel guilty accepting help from others. Or they do not want to impose or trouble anybody else. Some may feel embarrassed or too proud to ask. Thus, it is not uncommon for caregivers to take on the responsibilities alone, without the help of others.

Over time, the responsibilities of caregiving can become overwhelming, especially as the loved one's needs increase. Thus, it is important for the caregiver to learn to accept help if it is available. Other family members can be a valuable support resource. Allowing one's children to become involved is one step, as sometimes one parent is even reluctant to accept offers from the children to assist with caring for the ailing parent. Relatives living in close proximity and who are able to help, even if just for a few hours, can be valuable. Other people to consider include close friends or church friends. Accepting their offers of support will help relieve some of the caregiving strain and allow the primary caregiver to function better the rest of the time.

If there are no immediate relatives available, as everyone's family circumstances are different, or if the living environment does not make it feasible to ask friends or neighbors, there are other resources available. The local senior center or elder services organization may be able to provide volunteers who can help for a few hours. Home aides or companions may be available at subsidized costs. The local Alzheimer's association is also a good resource for finding someone who can help relieve the caregiver, if not regularly, at least occasionally.

## Adult Day Care

Besides finding someone to come to the home to help relieve the caregiver, another option is adult day care. Adult day care centers, sometimes referred to as adult day health centers, are facilities where persons with impairments such as dementia can go for several hours a day. They provide socialization and stimulation that they otherwise would not receive at home. Some facilities have programs specifically for persons with Alzheimer's disease. Some even provide pickup and drop-off service. They typically have scheduled activities aimed at promoting physical and emotional well-being of the participants through activities such as arts and crafts, music, and exercise classes.

Although adult day care is beneficial for both the person with Alzheimer's disease and his caregiver, it is not suitable for everyone. It would not be recommended for someone with advanced stages of Alzheimer's disease. But someone who is in the mild to moderate stages may benefit from the social stimulation and be able to participate in the activities. The facility will usually screen to determine whether a person is suitable for their program.

In addition to providing respite care, many adult day care centers also have support groups for the caregivers. They may also have social workers or counselors who are experienced in working with families of Alzheimer's patients and can provide support to caregivers as well. Furthermore, they are familiar with available services that may be beneficial, such as in-home help or financial assistance.

### In-Home Help

As Alzheimer's disease advances, the affected individual's needs become greater. The person may be able to live alone in the early stages, with someone checking in on a regular basis. If the individual lives with a spouse or child, he may be able to function without much assistance from them. However, as the memory and cognitive impairments worsen, he will need more assistance with his daily activities. It may get to the point where the spouse or child is unable to manage alone. It may be necessary to have someone come in to help. Local elder service agencies may be able to send in a home aide to help with light household chores, such as doing the laundry or vacuuming, for a few hours a week. They can also provide personal-care attendants who can help with grooming, such as bathing and getting dressed. If deemed necessary, these services are usually of no cost to the recipient. The limitation of these home services is that they are usually provided for only a few hours, up to a few times a week, depending on the needs of the individual.

When nursing needs arise, many communities have a visiting nurse agency that can make house calls. If there is a medical need, a physician can prescribe home visits by a nurse. Some services that a nurse can provide in the home setting include medication management, monitoring of certain medical conditions, and wound care. Having a nurse come to the home can be a great source of support for the caregiver. The nurse can also teach the caregiver to manage the affected person's medical conditions. In addition, it is a good way for the person's condition to be monitored closely, as the nurse keeps the physician updated on any changes. The nurse can also arrange for other services if necessary.

Nursing is not the only skilled services available through home health agencies. Rehabilitation can be provided by a physical therapist, occupational therapist, or speech therapist depending on the needs of the individual. For example, if the person's gait becomes increasingly unsteady, a physical therapist can work with him to try to walk better. The physical therapist can also fit him for a gait assistive device, such as a walker or cane, if necessary. If the person starts having difficulty with self-care such as grooming or eating, an occupational therapist can help. An occupational therapist can help with compensatory strategies based on the person's deficits, such as teaching the caregiver ways to simplify tasks for the person. The occupational therapist can also recommend adaptive equipment to modify the living environment to make it safer and optimal for the person's needs.

### Assisted Living

In some communities, there are apartment buildings or complexes called assisted living facilities. As the name suggests, an assisted living facility is for people who need some assistance with daily self-care activities but do not need constant supervision. The person would live in his own apartment but with someone coming in to help with bathing or assistance with medications. Meals may be provided in the building. However, there is no skilled nursing provided. This type of environment may be suitable for someone in the early stage of Alzheimer's disease. For someone who is no longer able to live independently but is still able to perform some self-care needs, moving to an assisted living building may be feasible.

### Skilled Nursing

Even with the available community resources, the time may come when a few hours of assistance a day may no longer be enough. The caregiver may need to hire someone to come for more hours than provided by home health agencies. The main complicating factor is usually cost, as it can become quite expensive to pay out of pocket for a health aide. Thus, it is important to plan financially early on and anticipate the costs. However, for many people, hiring help is not a feasible option.

As Alzheimer's disease progresses into the advanced stage, the individual's needs may overwhelm the caregiver. It may get to the point where the caregiver cannot handle it alone, such as if the person is wandering or aggressive. When the person becomes incontinent and eventually bedbound, it may be too much for one person to manage alone. A frail elderly woman may be unable to lift her husband to change him or transfer him in and out of bed. If he were to fall, she may not be strong enough to help him up.

Even with the best intentions, caring for someone with severe Alzheimer's disease can become too overwhelming. The time may come when around-the-clock skilled nursing is necessary. The topic of a nursing home is not an easy one to discuss. For many people, it is a difficult, even heart-wrenching, decision to make. It is not uncommon to be wracked with guilt if the decision is made to move a loved one with advanced Alzheimer's disease into a nursing home. But it is a necessary move if the person needs more care than can be provided at home.

Some nursing homes have a unit set aside for Alzheimer's disease or other dementias. These units are designed to promote optimal function and safety for persons with Alzheimer's disease. The staff is trained to work with their needs.

The transition to a long-term-care facility can be difficult for both the person and his caregiver. Even if the caregiver is no longer providing direct care, he or she continues to play an important role in the loved one's life. Besides making frequent visits, the caregiver will be updated on the loved one's condition regularly and will be consulted on any issues that arise. The caregiver will likely be called upon to make decisions regarding medical care as well.

# 8

# Scientific and Clinical Research in Alzheimer's Disease

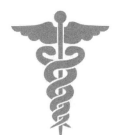

E ven though Alzheimer's disease was first described almost 100 years ago, there is still much that we do not know about the disease. As the aging population increases, so does the number of people who are diagnosed with Alzheimer's disease. Thus, there is an urgency to better understand the disease and develop better treatment options. There is much ongoing research into many aspects of Alzheimer's disease.

Many scientists are working hard to identify the cause of the disease and understand the disease process better. Researchers are also developing innovative diagnostic techniques to detect the disease earlier. Furthermore, researchers are trying to develop better medications to treat the symptoms of Alzheimer's disease. Medications to modify the disease, such as halting or reversing the disease process, are also being looked at. A way to prevent Alzheimer's disease, such as a vaccination, has also been proposed. Thus, there is a wealth of exciting research being conducted related Alzheimer's disease.

## DIAGNOSTIC TOOLS

Scientists are examining different ways to diagnose Alzheimer's disease. By the time a person exhibits signs, the brain changes have probably been taking place for years. The hope is to detect it before an individual shows any signs of dementia, and hopefully, be able to start treating it earlier. Some researchers are trying to develop a way to detect Alzheimer's by a simple blood or body fluid test. Others are examining new brain imaging techniques.

### Biomarkers

A biomarker is a substance or characteristic that can be objectively measured and is an indicator of a normal body process, disease process, or response to treatment. In Alzheimer's disease, the search is for biomarkers that are indicative of onset or presence of the disease process. So the hope is that with a blood or spinal fluid test, the presence of Alzheimer's disease can be detected early on, hopefully long before it becomes apparent to the patient and the caregiver. Many potential biomarkers are being studied, including proteins, antibodies, and inflammatory markers (Craig-Shapiro 2009). Most have not panned out, but there are a few that are promising, including two biomarkers in the cerebral spinal fluid, tau protein and CSF Ab42. These two biomarkers are reflective of amyloid deposition in the brain. However, spinal fluid is not as easily or routinely obtained as blood. Although there is still much work needed before a biomarker in blood is identified that is accurate and available as a diagnostic tool, it may not be that far off.

### Neuroimaging

We know today that Alzheimer's disease can start as early as 10 to 15 years before it can be diagnosed by our current methods. Neuroimaging has the potential to identify early changes in the brain and therefore potentially allow for an earlier diagnosis and treatment.

Traditionally, imaging modalities such at CT and MRI are used to evaluate brain changes associated with Alzheimer's disease. More recently, new neuroimaging modalities have been investigated that one day may potentially replace current imaging techniques. Functional MRIs and PET scans are promising imaging techniques that might aid in early diagnosis of Alzheimer's disease.

Functional MRI is different from traditional MRI in that it detects changes in blood flow related to neuronal activity. In addition to displaying brain structures, it generates images that reflect which structures become activated during the performance of tasks. The individual is shown different images, smells, or sounds while the MRI is performed. In Alzheimer's disease, decreased activity is usually seen in the temporal lobes and hippocampus, as well as other parts of the brain (Wierenga 2007). Researchers are looking at ways to improve this imaging technique and to apply this technology to diagnosis Alzheimer's disease more accurately and earlier in the disease process.

PET (positron emission tomography) scan is another type of neuroimaging technology. PET scans measure radioactively labeled chemical compounds injected into the bloodstream, which eventually travel to the brain. Brain activity, in the form of blood flow, oxygen, and glucose metabolism, is measured by the PET scanner. The multicolored images obtained depict the various areas of metabolic activity depending on the task. Decreased activity in certain areas, such as the hippocampus, can be suggestive of Alzheimer's disease. PET scans are potentially useful in that decreased activity in certain areas of the brain may be picked up early in the disease, when structure abnormalities or atrophy are not visualized yet. This imaging technique is being used more frequently, although it is not widely available yet.

## TREATMENT

For many, one of the most frustrating aspects of Alzheimer's disease is the lack of available therapy to halt the disease or reverse the damage. There is a lot of activity in this area of Alzheimer's research. Similar to the currently available medications are the drugs that can slow the decline but do not alter the actual disease process. Perhaps what is more exciting are the drugs that can potentially stop the degenerative process.

The process of developing a drug, from conception to animal studies to human trials to approval for public use, is a long and arduous one. It can take decades, and many drugs do not pan out as hoped. Thus, the drugs currently in development that will be discussed below may eventually fail clinical or safety trials and never become available to the public.

### Dimebon

Dimebon is a drug that may slow cognitive decline in people with mild to moderate Alzheimer's disease (Doody 2008). It is believed to prevent neuronal death by stabilizing the mitochondria, a cell structure important in energy production. It may also have an effect on acetylcholine esterase and NMDA receptors, which are involved in memory (Bachurin 2001). This experimental drug is currently in phase III clinical trials in the United States. This means that it is being tested in a large group of people, up to 3,000, to evaluate its effectiveness, side effects, and any safety issues. There are several clinical trials for dimebon currently being conducted or enrolling participants, looking at effectiveness in all stages of Alzheimer's disease. Unfortunately, recent results from one of the clinical trials showed that dimebon may not be more effective than a placebo in treating patients with Alzheimer's disease (http://investors. medivation.com/ releasedetail.cfm?ReleaseID=448818). However, the drug maker Pfizer is still running several other trials with this medication, and the results are still pending.

### Bapineuzumab

Bapineuzumab is a drug that acts as an antibody to beta-amyloids. Antibodies are proteins in the body that protect it from invading foreign objects such as bacteria. They are produced in response to the particular attacker, or antigen. Bapineuzumab is a monoclonal antibody, meaning it is developed to selectively attack beta-amyloids and reduce beta-amyloid accumulation in the brain. A study with a small group of participants demonstrated potential benefits that warrant further investigation (Salloway 2009). Enrollment of participants is currently underway for phase III clinical trials, the results of which should be published within the next few years.

### IVIG

IVIG (intravenous immunoglobulin) is being considered as a potential treatment for Alzheimer's disease. IVIG is a blood product consisting of antibodies, or immunoglobulins, extracted from pooled donor blood. It is administered intravenously, or directly into the bloodstream. It contains naturally occurring antibodies that act against amyloid. One study suggested that previous treatment with IVIG was associated with a reduced risk of Alzheimer's disease (Fillit 2009). Thus, a phase III clinical trial is currently underway to better study the effects of IVIG on Alzheimer's disease, with preliminary data estimated to become available in 2011.

### Semagacestat

Semagacestat is a gamma-secretase inhibitor. Drugs that can inhibit or modulate gamma-secretase are of great interest in Alzheimer's drug development. Gamma-secretase is the pivotal enzyme that generates beta-amyloid. Thus, if one can prevent gamma-secretase from working properly, it may be possible to reduce beta-amyloid production. Other gamma-secretase inhibitors in the past have been unsuccessful, and there were some concerns about potential toxicity. Clinical trials for semagacestat are currently being conducted to further assess its efficacy and safety.

### Targeting Tau

In addition to anti-amyloid therapy, researchers are also trying to develop drugs that target tau proteins. Abnormal tau aggregation leads to eventual formation of neurofibrillary tangles, which are pathologic features of Alzheimer's disease. Methylene blue, a widely used dye to study cells, is thought to possibly interfere with tau aggregation. Plans are underway for it to be studied on a larger scale (Rafii 2009). Unlike anti-amyloid therapy, the development of drugs that target tau currently lag behind development of drugs aimed at beta-amyloids.

At the Alzheimer's Association's 2010 International Conference on Alzheimer's Disease (AAICAD 2010) in Honolulu, four new very preliminary research studies were presented which described experimental immunotherapies targeting the tau protein. A gene called FTO has been identified that may increase the risk of developing Alzheimer's disease, especially if the person also carries the ApoE gene. The use of intranasal insulin is being studied for possible benefits in Alzheimer's disease ( http://www.alz.org/icad/). Stem cell–based therapy has been considered for neurodegenerative disease such as Alzheimer's disease, but it is unclear at this point whether it is feasible (Lindvall 2010). Furthermore, groups of experts are working to update the diagnostic criteria for Alzheimer's disease, which will hopefully lead to earlier diagnosis and treatment (http://www.alz.org/icad/2010_release_diagnostic_071310_130pm.asp).

These are some examples of therapies and new strategies currently being developed in the treatment of Alzheimer's disease. Some of these may possibly become available in the near future. There are many other technologies and drugs that may be on the horizon. The future direction of Alzheimer's disease is to better understand the causes, make an earlier diagnosis, and develop more effective therapies.

While we wait for better treatments or even a cure, many scientists are also looking at how to prevent the disease in the first place. Is it preventable? The short answer is, we don't know at this time, but there is increasing evidence showing that it may be worthwhile trying. Over the last 20 years, numerous studies have been done to try to answer this question. Many of the trials were disappointing and resulted in conflicting results. However, there were some studies that may point us in the right direction. The current recommendations are the following:

- Vitamin E is not recommended for the treatment or prevention of Alzheimer's disease. There has been a lot of interest in the role of vitamins, especially antioxidants that act against toxic free radicals. Vitamin E was believed to be helpful at one point, but the data has been inconclusive

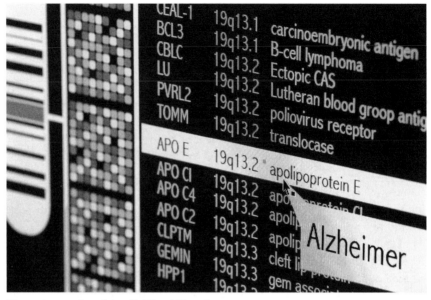

Genomic mapping of ApoE. (iStockPhoto)

since. Current guidelines do not recommend its use in Alzheimer's disease (Isaac 2008).

- Gingko biloba has not been consistently shown to have benefits in dementia. Gingko biloba is an extract from the maidenhair tree, which has been used in China for centuries for many ailments. It is frequently touted in the media and used by many people for memory problems. However, the studies conducted to date have not demonstrated conclusively its favorable effects on memory (Birks 2009).

- Hormone replacement therapy is not recommended. Female hormone replacement was once proposed as a possible treatment to prevent memory and cognitive decline. Studies have not supported this theory, and in fact, have demonstrated potentially life-threatening side effects including increased risk of heart attacks and strokes (Hogervorst 2009) (Rapp 2003).

- Nonsteroidal anti-inflammatory drugs (NSAIDs) are not recommended for the prevention of Alzheimer's disease. NSAIDs, such as ibuprofen and aspirin, are commonly used as pain-relievers and are readily available at drugstores. Early studies have suggested potential protective benefits, but later studies did not show a positive effect (Imbimbo 2009).

- Omega-3 fatty acids, or fish oil, may not decrease dementia risk. Of the studies conducted to date, some have suggested benefits, but these positive results have not been confirmed by other data (Devore 2009). However, moderate fish consumption as part of a well-balanced diet can contribute to maintaining health.

- Cholesterol-lowering medications, called statins, are not recommended for the treatment of Alzheimer's disease at this time. Some data have suggested a possible reduced risk of dementia, but a recent study did not find it to slow the cognitive decline in people with Alzheimer's disease (Feldman 2010).

- No particular diet has been shown to prevent dementia. Nonetheless, a well-balanced diet rich in fruits and vegetables is key to promoting good health. Some studies suggest a potential benefit on memory and cognition in following a Mediterranean-type diet, which emphasizes fruits, nuts, vegetables, and healthy fats such as olive oil (Féart 2009) (Scarmeas 2009).

- Physical exercise and keeping socially and mentally engaged are important aspects of maintaining overall and brain health. These activities may not prevent the onset of dementia, but they can potentially delay its development (Lautenschlager 2008). A recent study suggests that increased physical activity may reduce of risk of Alzheimer's disease (Scarmeas 2009). Although more data is needed, regular physical exercise, social and mental engagement, in addition to a well-balanced diet, are essential ingredients to one's well-being.

# Appendix A

## Narratives

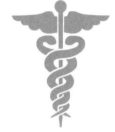

### MILLIE'S STORY

This is my perspective on what it's like to have Alzheimer's disease. To begin with, to me Alzheimer's disease is an insidious disease. It creeps up on you. My wife, Mildred, showed evidence of some memory problems years ago. She's 77 years old now. But she was 65 when she started having these problems. She would forget short-term events. She would think I had told her something when I didn't. Or I would tell her something myself but she didn't remember it. And all these memory tricks went on continuously. Now, Millie used to work at a girls' private high school. And Millie was very good with computers and she would set up the computer program for the entire school, which had 400 students. But there were times when this was in place, and Millie was making mistakes on the computer. It wasn't like her at all. She was very efficient. Unfortunately, I didn't know about this until after she retired. Millie always took good care of herself. She had a physical exam every year. And at one point, when I saw this condition manifest itself, I wrote a letter to her physician explaining what I was seeing and letting him know what was happening. He made all kinds of preliminary tests. When he saw her, he tested her for B12 deficiency. He gave her an MRI. All these pointed to Alzheimer's disease.

At the beginning of her sickness, things went fairly well. Millie was in a low-key situation. She would sit on the porch and just talk, relax. But, unfortunately, Alzheimer's is a progressive disease and you reach different plateaus. And Millie was on her way to reaching these plateaus. There came a time when Millie was very, very agitated. It seemed like she wanted to leave the house all the time. I had to lock the doors and keep the keys in my pocket. I had to physically stop her from going out the door. There were times at the beginning when I would go shopping for food and when I came home, she would be gone. She would be walking the neighborhood. This was a very disturbing situation. Millie continually got worse in her situation and she seemed to reach different plateaus. And these plateaus would come without warning. She would continually walk through the house, wanting to get out. And this went on through the night. She would get up out of bed and want to leave. I understand that they have a feeling that they want to go back home. Millie would be on her feet all day long and all night. And her feet started to swell.

It was suggested that Millie go to a day care for Alzheimer's. So we made arrangements for her to go to an Alzheimer's day care. This was under the direction of a psychiatrist that we had consulted for Millie. Millie was still ambulatory at this point. And also cognitive of what was happening. But Millie was so used to working in this girls' high school that she was sort of the assistant to the principal. And when she went to the Alzheimer's day care, she took it on herself to be the assistant of the resident nurse there. So she would prevent people from going into the nurse's office. And they had to call me and tell me that something had to be done or she couldn't stay there. She was stopping people from seeing the nurse. It seemed to be her role to keep order in an organization. Millie continued to slow down and she would reach different plateaus. There came a point when Millie refused to go to the day care. She used to be picked up by a small bus. So there came a time when she didn't want to go anymore and she'd refuse to go down the stairs. Stairs caused a big problem for Millie, so that was another plateau she was on.

There came a time when I couldn't take care of all of Millie's needs by myself. And I had to recruit health care aides. So I started with a health care aide in the morning to give Millie a bath, when Millie was still ambulatory. So the health care aide and I would park Millie from one room to another. This went on for maybe six months. And all of a sudden, Millie couldn't walk anymore so she stayed in bed. She's been bedridden now for two years. She's not able to feed herself although she does have a good appetite. She cannot feed herself, she has to be fed. I would get Millie up every morning and place her in her wheelchair and wheel her to a lounge chair in another room. And have her sit for two to three hours and relax. And I'd get her back to bed again. This seems to be helpful for her general condition.

But as time went on, Millie didn't recognize me or our children. We have three girls. She doesn't recognize our children. And at this stage, Millie is completely bedridden except for two to three hours sitting on a lounge chair in the morning. She's not able to help herself at all. She still has a good appetite. Millie has to be fed every meal. Millie had been taking Aricept throughout her illness. At this point, the Aricept didn't help at all so we stopped giving it to her. Millie was also on Seroquel and this calmed her down dramatically. Unfortunately, she gained weight taking this medication. So when Millie was strictly bedridden, we stopped Seroquel and she's been calm ever since.

At the beginning, I mentioned that I felt Alzheimer's was an insidious disease and it has many ramifications. It seems like the medical profession considers Alzheimer's as a done deal, where nothing can be done about it. But I think a lot of the things that are not life-threatening that happen to an Alzheimer's patient should be addressed. It reminds me of this person who had a large grocery store and he had live lobsters at his store. He was very particular about taking good care of these lobsters. And someone said to him, "How come you're so particular about these lobsters when people are going to kill them and eat them anyway?" And he says, "As long as they are living, they should be respected and made comfortable." That's how I feel about Alzheimer's patients. I think, in general, the medical profession seems to consider it a done deal, that nothing can be done about it. It doesn't seem to be worth the time and effort. There are things that happen to Alzheimer's patients that happen to everyone else. They get skin rashes and things like that; it would be nice to address them. Right now, Millie is doing fairly well. She sleeps quite a bit of the time. Never complains. When she's awake, she seems like she can be alert.

This is my understanding of Alzheimer's disease. It's really a subjective view of it rather than an objective view, and I don't think I can view it any differently. As I think back at the beginning of Millie's sickness, she was sitting on the porch with me and she asked me a question that was tough to answer. She said, "Is there something wrong with me?" That took me back a bit and I said, "No, nothing wrong. You just have a little trouble with your memory." We never did tell Millie that she has Alzheimer's disease. In retrospect, I think I would like to know myself if I had it. It seems like a tough thing to tell somebody. A strange thing just happened recently. Our home health aide has a loud voice and a loud laugh, and she always talks to Millie when she's bathing her. She tells her about her experiences and things like that. And Millie seems to be listening to it. She said that Millie looked so great she had a great swagger, and Millie, after two years without saying a word, repeated the word "swagger." It was a surprise.

It's a tough situation to be a so-called caregiver for an Alzheimer's patient because you have feelings of guilt and paranoia. You want to do as much as you can for them, and you don't want them to feel abandoned. The bottom line is, it's very tough. Besides trying to cope with the Alzheimer's, we still have to cope with the everyday trial and tribulations of running a household, trying to rectify things that go wrong, say with the furnace and things like that, and trying to keep the house clean.

—Jack

## A WIFE'S STORY

It was about seven years ago that I first noticed a change in my husband's memory. He will repeatedly ask me questions. This was before I realized what was happening. The biggest thing was his driving. He was always a cautious driver. However, he started to drive on the right side of the freeway, where the cars go to get off on the ramp. If I said anything to him, he would say he's been driving his whole life and he knew how to drive. The next thing I noticed was, when we would go to our children's house, it was an awful ride. He was going very, very slowly. I used to say, he wouldn't be in an accident but he would cause an accident. One day, we came off the Mass Pike going toward our daughter's home; he should have of taken a right but he asked me which way to go. He didn't know where we were going. That shocked me. He had been driving there many times. He used to drive our daughter, who was a nurse, into the city to Brigham and Women's Hospital. She would notice different things on the ride in. Our son, a police officer, he noticed things as well. My husband owned his own real estate business. Our oldest daughter worked in his office and noticed changes in him as well.

He would never let me go to the doctor with him. I spoke with his doctor about my concerns, and he went to a neurologist. That was when he was diagnosed. He couldn't remember what day it was. He would say "What's today?" He got sick in May 2007 and was taken out of the house by ambulance. He had an infection in the spine. His memory got worse in the hospital. He was in the intensive care unit for several weeks. Eventually, he did come home.

Right now, he's progressing very quickly in terms of the short-term memory loss. He can't remember the day or the year. Yesterday, we went to Mass. He didn't remember any of that. He sits and reads the paper for hours. He doesn't go to the office every day anymore. He can't remember whether he went or not. He goes and reads the paper. Sometimes he'll read the paper from the day before. I will drop him off at the office after Mass. He's usually at the office all day, unless he gets tired.

He seems to sleep an awful lot. He showers and shaves himself. There are times when I'll say, "Did you take a shower?" He'll say "I did." "Did you wash your hair?" "I don't remember." He's always been a neat dresser, in a suit daily. Now, he doesn't change his shirts. I'll set out his slacks and socks. He doesn't change his slacks.

He still has a sense of humor. He will tell the kids about when he first walked me home from a school dance. We'll be married 54 years in September. He'll talk about things in the past, from when he was a boy. But he can't remember whether he went to church today. It's the short- term memory that our children and I have noticed.

Driving was a big, big thing. No one was going to tell him not to drive. "I'm alright." My daughter has his car now. Every once in awhile, he'll ask where his car is. His license expired last year. My daughter checked with the Alzheimer's Association and they said they could take him out for a road test. He was very upset when my son took him in. Then we got a notice from the registry that his license would be suspended due to medical reasons. It was just last week that he said he wanted to get his license again. He got very angry when I explained why he couldn't drive. He hasn't mentioned for a few days now about getting his license back. He hasn't driven since last September, after he almost got us into an accident. He was swerving into a parked car. He was steering into other cars. He hasn't driven since.

He's very independent. He was one of 13, and he always said he took care of himself. That's how he was. He more or less did his own thing, whatever he wanted to. He still has his sense of humor.

He's great with the grandkids. He's always asking the grandkids how many boy-friends or girlfriends they have. They are patient with him. He's always asking them how old they are, what grade in school they are, even the ones in college. Five minutes later, he asks the same questions again. He'll ask me the same questions over and over again. "What month, date, year?" The grandkids do tell their parents that they see a change in him.

Once, while my son's two children were here, he said to me "Barbara, who are those kids in the living room?" When they were leaving and backing out of the driveway, he said to me "Barbara, who are those kids in the car?"

I've always given him his medications. I used to put them out on the table for him. One night, out of the blue, he said he won't take the pills. The next morning, he said I'm not going to take the pills anymore because they're not helping. They're giving me nightmares. What I have been doing since, I pull the Exelon capsule apart and put it in his cereal. I crush Namenda in his cereal and put more sugar in his raisin bran. He has the same cereal every morning. I asked the pharmacist and he said it was alright. But I can't get them into him at night. I think he's sleeping better at night because he's not taking them at night.

Some mornings he'll say to me after breakfast, "Barbara, I didn't eat breakfast." It's our routine to eat breakfast and go to Mass. Sometimes, he'll get tired and say, "I want to go home. I want to go home."

I would have to say that I have a lot of support from my children and grandchildren. I'm not kidding myself. I have two dear friends who had Alzheimer's disease, and they were different. They tell us at the meetings that no two people's Alzheimer's disease are alike. I say to my kids, it's only going to get worse. His sister has it as well, and she's further along. Thank goodness, physically, he seems to be doing well. Sometimes, he'll say "something's happening to my memory." He got upset when I mentioned Alzheimer's disease once.

The Alzheimer's Association has been wonderful. They are wonderful to talk to. One time, he locked himself out of the house. "I went out the driveway and I forgot why I was there." It hasn't happened since. The Alzheimer's Association suggested putting a lock way up on top. Day programs have been suggested, but honestly, I don't think he'll go.

We plan not to plan. There are times when he just doesn't want to do something. You have to just take one day at a time. There are good days and there are bad days. Take it one day at a time.

—Barbara

## AUNT E'S STORY

I have known Aunt E for 32 years and to be more accurate, Aunt E is my wife's aunt on her mother's side of the family. Aunt E is 86 years old. She was married for 28 years and has been a widow for over 30 years. She had no children. She was employed at Polaroid Corporation for over 25 years as an assembly line supervisor. In this position she had charge of 12 people, mostly women employees. This short biography I believe is important because it explains a particularly evident part of her past and present character: a desire for independence that she has cherished and has been able to maintain for her entire life. As an employed woman she supervised many employees and proudly still remembers and identifies with the supervisory role that she demonstrated for over 25 years and is now, in her own words: "a nobody." During her recollections of her employment and supervisory experience she often repeats only one or two specific stories from her employment history. I think the one story that gives credence to her need for independence is the recounting of the time that she needed to discipline an employee for some cause and when not supported by her executive managers decided to retire early. It seems that this demonstration of independence stays in her memory and is frequently repeated to us now needing no encouragement from us and often as a non sequitur in the conversation that is at hand. During and after her marriage, she traveled and completely enjoyed the company of family and friends. She was known to be particularly family oriented in that on special holidays such as July 4th, New Year's Day, she would invite the entire family (nephews and nieces, cousins, and sisters) to her home for either a home-cooked meal or an impromptu Chinese take-out dinner. She was very well-known in her family circle for providing a rich assortment of bake goods for any special family occasion. The home-baked treats were anticipated and welcomed. For many years she was known to provide transportation for neighbors and friends who could no longer walk or drive to local stores. For a short time she took up a part-time job to provide extra income for herself but also to have something to do with her time and to "get out of the house."

She was and still is very opinionated and has never been afraid to speak her mind. In some instances it seemed to me at least, that she would intentionally take a contrary viewpoint if only to present another opinion for the purpose of being allowed to express it. She was and is generous to charity causes, particularly those causes that involve animals such as animal shelters or the MSPCA (Massachusetts Society for the Prevention of Cruelty to Animals). Until recently she attended Catholic mass daily driving herself and a neighbor to the church. She also donated to the church where she would also meet many other neighbors and old friends.

In hindsight, I believe the first signs of diminished memory were when the quality of her home- baked treats started to degrade. An ingredient was left out or the baking time was not correct; something diminished the quality of the baked product. At the time, perhaps four or five years ago, this misstep was given little or no attention by the family. She would excuse the error as being caused by her "rushing to attend" the particular family get-together; an excuse that she still uses but now on a much more regular basis. If she has misplaced her house keys, puts on the wrong clothes for the season, or is not ready when you've arranged a time for her "pickup" for an appointment she "just doesn't like to be rushed." However, it became noticeable that she would bake less often until the baking stopped completely. She replaced the home-baked treats with baked foods purchased in local stores. But it is also important to note that during the last several years she has witnessed the loss of her sisters due to old age and ill health and thus there were fewer family celebratory occasions and overall less reason to celebrate in her own fashion.

About two years ago, she was involved in a small auto accident when she hit the door of a parked car when the driver of the parked auto opened the door "too quickly and she didn't see him with enough time to stop." Fortunately, no one was injured but her old and relatively large car was totaled. She insisted on having it replaced. Given the circumstances of the accident it did seem that the accident may not have been her fault (no claims were made against her by the other driver) and at the time there was no concern about her continuing to drive.

During the summer of 2009, we began to notice peculiarities in her demeanor and habits that caused us concern; enough concern to start watching her more carefully. For example, it seemed to us that there were many more of her tales of fast driving and being stopped by police officers with only "warnings." These stories were only told to us to give us some appreciation for her prowess in being able to convince the police officer that she was speeding only because "she needed to go to the bathroom" and therefore should not get a speeding ticket. However, some of these police stops were on streets that she did not have a very good reason for using given her normal shopping habits and venues. On occasions when we knew where she was going and therefore had some idea of when to expect her home at a certain hour it seemed that she would take much longer for her to complete her errands. On one remarkable occasion, for example, she was gone for five hours to a hairdresser's appointment in a town that is only seven miles away. She finally returned only to have her hair give clear proof that she had not been able to keep her appointment. She declared that she decided to "cancel the appointment for another time."

The watershed event that confirmed for us that her memory was, in fact, impaired was her failure to pay important bills such as her home insurance and utility bills. In one instance we actually found her arguing on the phone with an insurance agent who told us that an insurance payment was two months late and yet Aunt E insisted that she did send them a payment. On another occasion when her phone was "out of order" we discovered that the utility had shut off service for lack of payment. An immediate call to the utility restored service, with apologies, when they were told that she was elderly. Since then all bills are being paid by my wife but with Aunt E's written permission. In September 2009 we took the car away from her. From September until today, my wife provides transportation to and from shopping centers, the hairdresser, church, the bank, to weeknight dinners at our house, etc. After taking the car away, her phone calls to our home increased to the point where the telephone message recorder identified as many as 65 calls in one day. The message was always the same: "Who has my car? I want it back in the drive way . . . I won't drive it . . . I feel more secure with it in the driveway." With each of the calls, which are sometimes only 5 to 10 minutes apart, the message that is left sounds as if it is being left for the first time; that is, with no reference to earlier messages or any annoyance on her part that previous messages have been ignored. It is also important to note that with the passing of all of her older sisters she no longer is able to phone them to engage in what were many daily, albeit brief, phone conversations. The sisters would engage themselves in these daily phone conversations throughout their lives and the absence of this ritual must now be very distressing to Aunt E during the day when she is alone.

Aunt E continues to "want her car back," not knowing who has taken it and not realizing she hasn't had the vehicle for over six months. For example, the absence of the car each morning is blamed on someone having borrowed it the night before and not having returned it. She still insists that she alone will know when she cannot safely drive the car. She denies adamantly that she has ever had an accident or that her doctor has judged her to be incompetent to drive safely. She needs to be constantly reminded that her license has expired and believes this only when she checks the expiration date on her license.

During her meals with us, she will join in on the conversations, but she does have a constant refrain that reminds us that "this is too much of a bother for you to have me here for dinner" and "next weekend I want everyone to come to my house for dinner." It is clear to us that she does not know she is repeating herself. However, dinnertime is also a time when she recalls many things of her childhood with her sisters, mom, and dad, and regales us with specific stories. She still remembers many words and phrases in Italian—a language that she did not much use after her marriage—but often it becomes clear that she does not recall the meaning of some of the words that she is using. She also still remembers the names of deceased actors and actresses who may appear on an old (1940s and 1950s) movie that might be playing on the cable station. And she is still alert enough to understand when you are "trying to change the subject" in an attempt to stop her from asking "who has my car? I want it back in the driveway." However, when the TV sets were recently changed from analog to digital signal requiring a different "on and off" control, she cannot remember how to use the new TV controls.

The memory lapses as evidenced by specific events are no longer surprising to us now, but we are surprised by how quickly her memory has declined. It is only heartening to realize that any reason that she thinks she has for becoming annoyed with us for not giving her what she wants or for constantly reminding her of her next appointment as if "she were a child . . . because . . . I'm not senile yet you know," is a memory that disappears quickly. She is thus not burdened by the past, inferred grievances, and her personality upon the next encounter still remains the "old" Aunt E and she greets us without recalling any perceived grievance. It is sad however, to realize that her admonition to us that "I'm not senile yet you know" is offered more and more frequently and is, I believe, an indication that she does in fact realize that something is missing; that all is not the same as before. I believe she is becoming aware of a memory problem . . . if only for a rational moment . . . when it is gently demonstrated to her that she has been to the bank today as evidence of a bank envelope filled with money, or she has been to the hairdresser today as evidenced by a new hair style that she is wearing, or that she has had supper over at our house today as evidenced by leftovers in her refrigerator, or that she has been to church as evidence of the palms she has brought home from Palm Sunday services, or that she has fed the dog today as evidenced by the dirty dog dish. It is sadder still to think that these "rational moments" are causing her more distress than relief.

## A DAUGHTER'S PERSPECTIVE

It started about 10 years ago: my mother who has always prided herself on her organizational skills and mathematic abilities all of a sudden found herself having difficulty organizing and paying her bills. She would look at her checkbook and not remember how to complete the check, how to log it, and whether or not she paid a bill. Along with this, she and I noticed that at times she had difficulty making sense of numbers and difficulty expressing her thoughts. She would say I know the word but I can't say it . . . First we thought, is this some new medication that is causing this trouble? Could she have an infection or be having small strokes? A visit to the primary care doctor and neurologist proved that neither one of these things was happening. Then there was a request for further evaluation and testing to rule out Alzheimer's disease.

I remembered thinking at this time that if it is Alzheimer's disease she will probably be fine with medication, and then the start of denial was on its way. Alzheimer's disease as we know is a progressive disease with no cure. As a nurse I was quite aware of that; as a daughter I was sure that this progression would not happen to my mother. As her disease progressed and it did, despite medications, I saw my mother change before my eyes. At first, I became angry. Is she on the right medication? Isn't there anything anyone can do? Is enough being done? There must be something and we are missing it. Once I read about some sophisticated testing in one of the magazines that may help and was sure this was the answer. Of course it was not. After that came the sadness, the loss of my relationship as I know it with my mother. The changes in the way she experienced life and relationships with her grandchildren and my brother.

I realized that I kept focusing on the things she could no longer do and not the things she could. With support from my good friends, I started talking about the changes with friends and my family. When I looked at my mother and saw she was happy, she was smiling. She was not worried about what she could not remember. She actually could enjoy the day. It was then I decided to emphasize and celebrate the things she could do and let go of the things she couldn't. And so although Mom at times did not know my name or really could not tell someone who I was, I knew she loved me because her face lit up every time she saw me. She knew I loved her and was always happy to see me. We could enjoy many things together. It may not be the baseball game because she could not follow it anymore, but it was a beautiful spring day looking at flowers or laughing about something funny she said.

One thing that really helped my children, my brother, and me was to mirror her reality. And to go along with her conversations, and when we did, we found our connection with her during this time. My mom passed away on June 23, 2009. She had all her children and grandchildren with her at the time of her passing. Although she would not have been able to tell you our names, we know that she knew us as hers and that she knew we loved her and we knew she loved us.

# Appendix B

## Timeline

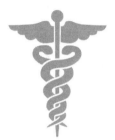

1864    Alois Alzheimer was born on June 14 in Marktbreit, a small Bavarian village near the town of Wuerzburg in southern Germany.

1887    Alois received his medical degree from the university of Wuerzburg.

1888    Dr. Alois Alzheimer started his medical career at the Hospital for Mentally Ill and Epileptics in Frankfurt am Main.

1894    Dr. Alzheimer married Mrs. Caecilie Geisenhammer with whom he had three children. Caecilie died unexpectedly in 1901.

1895    Dr. Alzheimer was appointed the director of the local Asylum for Lunatics and Epileptics in Frankfurt.

1903    After the death of his wife, Dr. Alzheimer left for Munich to join Emil Kraepelin, who was considered one of the most prominent psychiatrists.

1904    Dr. Alzheimer published results on a large study of general paralysis of the insane. This was to become one of Alzheimer's best-known works in which he correlated histological findings with clinical presentation of the disease.

1906    At a meeting of the superintendents of mental asylums in Germany, Dr. Alzheimer presented a paper on the "peculiar disease of the cerebral cortex." In the paper he described the case study of a patient at the Frankfurt asylum named Auguste D., whom he had followed closely until her death that same year. He compared the clinical and histopathological findings of the brain biopsy and described unknowingly the first documented case of a particular dementia which later carried his name.

1910    Dr. Emil Kraeplin proposed that the disease first described by his friend and colleague be named after Alzheimer himself.

1912    King Wilhelm II of Prussia approved the appointment of Dr. Alzheimer as a full professor of psychiatry at the university of Breslau (now Poland).

1915    Dr. Alzheimer died at the age of 51 on December 19 in Breslau, never having actually taken up his duties at the university because of a progressively worsening heart condition. He is buried in Frankfurt am Main.

1960's    Scientists discovered a relationship between cognitive decline and the amount of tangles and plaques in the brain of patients suffering from a dementia.

1970's    Alzheimer's disease gained popularity and was found to be present more often in patients with dementia.

1980    The Alzheimer's Disease and Related Disorders Association was incorporated. Today it is known as the Alzheimer's Association with headquarters in Chicago, Illinois.

1982    President Ronald Regan designated the first National Alzheimer's Disease Awareness Week.

1984    Alzheimer's Disease International (ADI) was founded.

1986    The Alois Alzheimer Center opened in Cincinnati, Ohio. This was the first specialized facility specializing in the care and study of patients suffering from Alzheimer's disease.

1990    The first FDA-approved drug, Cognex, was used to try to slow the progression of the disease.

1994    September 21 was launched as World Alzheimer's Day.

1995    Psychiatrists rediscovered Auguste Deter's medical records in the archives of the University of Frankfurt. These included the original admission report and handwritten notes by Dr. Alzheimer himself.

2006    Centenary year of Alzheimer's disease.

2010    Alzheimer's Disease International estimated 36.5 million people living worldwide with dementia in 2010 and 115.4 million people by 2050.

# Appendix C

## 10 Useful Web Sites

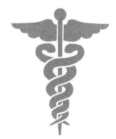

The following are some useful Web sites for further information about Alzheimer's disease. There are an overwhelming number of Web sites on this topic but these sites listed below provide a high quality of the information. Please note that these Web sites may change over time. At the time this book was published the information below was accurate.

### 1. WWW.ALZ.ORG

The Alzheimer's Association is a national organization whose mission is to "help fight Alzheimer's disease through vital research and essential support programs and services." The Web site is easy to navigate and provides excellent information on Alzheimer's disease under the Alzheimer's disease tab. For information on other dementias, use the "Related Dementias" field under the Alzheimer's disease tab. Caregivers can find helpful information by clicking on the "Living with Alzheimer's" tab.

### 2. WWW.ALZ.CO.UK

The Web site of Alzheimer's Disease International is very informative and provides excellent information on international activities around the research and statistics of Alzheimer's disease worldwide. The "I have dementia" tab at the top of the home page provides detailed steps for patients and their caregivers after the diagnosis of a dementia.

### 3. WWW.ALZFDN.ORG

The Alzheimer's Foundation of America is the main competitor of the Alzheimer's Association. The Web site is easy to navigate and well organized. The "Helpful links" section in the lower left part of the home page is particularly informative.

### 4. WWW.CAREGIVER.ORG

This Web site of the Family Caregiver Alliance provides excellent information for caregivers on a local, regional, and state level. It is referred to as a "one-stop shopping center for caregivers." The Web site also offers some information fact sheets in both Spanish and Chinese.

### 5. WWW.CDC.GOV

The official Web site of the Centers for Disease Control and Prevention is a useful place to start a search on many topics on aging including Alzheimer's disease. Just enter the word "aging" in the search field, and then look under the section "Learn More About. . . ."

### 6. WWW.HEALTHINAGING.ORG

This is the Web site for the Foundation of Health in Aging, a nonprofit organization founded by the American Geriatrics Society (AGS) in 1999. Enter dementia or Alzheimer's disease in the search field on the upper right corner of the home page. This will provide the reader with up-to-date information on the topic. Family caregivers will find useful information when clicking on the "Eldercare at Home" tab.

### 7. WWW.ICAREVILLAGE.COM

This relatively new Web site on "everything eldercare" offers a novel and easy way to navigate through a vast array of information. Clicking on the different tabs will provide good and helpful information, ranging from specific disease descriptions to caregiver, legal, and financial advice. The "Ask the Experts" tab will provide videos and encourages questions.

## 8. WWW.MAYOCLINIC.COM

This is a very useful and easy Web site to navigate. Under the heading of "Diseases and Conditions," you can search for information on a disease by clicking on its first letter. The disease descriptions are precise, up-to-date, and written in easy-to-understand language.

## 9. WWW.NCCAM.NIH.GOV

This is the official Web site of the National Center for Complementary and Alternative Medicine (NCCAM). The best way to start browsing this site is to click on the "A–Z Index of Health Topics" tab. The information on herbal and other complementary medicinal approaches is scientific and honest.

## 10. WWW.NIA.NIH.GOV

This is the Web site of the U.S. National Institutes of Health, featuring the National Institute on Aging. The tabs "Alzheimer's Disease Information" and "NIHSeniorHealth.gov" are very useful. The tabs are under the heading "Health Information."

# Glossary

**Aceytcholine:** A neurotransmitter that plays an important role in the nervous system.

**Agnosia:** Loss of ability to recognize familiar objects, persons, or sounds.

**Amygdala:** An almond-shaped structure located in the temporal lobe that processes and stores strong emotions.

**Amyloid plaque:** Protein fragments that build up between nerve cells in the brain, originating from amyloid precursor proteins.

**Apraxia:** Loss of ability to carry out learned, purposeful movements.

**Axon:** A long extension from the cell body that transmits signals or messages to other cells.

**Cerebral cortex:** The outer layer of the cerebral hemispheres.

**Delusion:** A false belief that is resistant to reason or evidence to the contrary.

**Dementia:** A general term used to describe the loss of memory and mental abilities severe enough to affect daily life.

**Dendrite:** An extension of the cell body that receives signals from other cells.

**Executive function:** The ability to organize, carry out thoughts and activities, prioritize tasks, and make decisions.

**Frontal lobe:** Located at the front of the brain, it is the part of the cerebral cortex involved in executive function—planning, organizing, problem solving.

**Glutamate:**  A neurotransmitter that plays an important role in learning and memory.

**Hallucination:**  Perception of images or sounds without an actual external stimulus.

**Hippocampus:**  Located in the temporal lobe, it is a key structure involved in formation and storage of memory.

**Mild cognitive impairment:**  A condition in which a person has problems with memory and mental abilities that are noticeable and detected on tests but are not significant enough to interfere with daily life.

**Neurofibrillary tangle:**  Bundle of twisted and tangled fibers inside nerve cells, mostly made of abnormal tau proteins.

**Neuron:**  A brain or nerve cell.

**Neurotransmitter:**  Chemical messenger between neurons. It is released by the axon and travels across the synapse to the receiving dendrite.

**Occipital lobe:**  Part of the cerebral cortex involved in vision.

**Parietal lobe:**  Part of the cerebral cortex involved in perception and sensation.

**Placebo:**  A sham pill that does not contain actual medicinal properties.

**Side effect:**  An undesirable effect caused by a medication in addition to its intended use.

**Synpase:**  A tiny gap between axon and dendrite across which neurotransmitters travel.

**Tardive dyskinesia:**  Muscle movements that a person cannot control. Often occurs as a result of taking antipsychotic medications.

**Tau:**  A protein that stabilizes microtubules in normal nerve cells.

**Temporal lobe:**  Part of the cerebral cortex involved in processing and storing memory.

# Bibliography

Altman, Lawrence. "The Doctor's World; A Recollection of Early Questions About Reagan's Health." *New York Times*, June 15, 2004. http://www.nytimes.com/2004/06/15/health/the-doctor-s-world-a-recollection-of-early-questions-about-reagan-s-health.html?sec=&spon=&pagewanted=all.

Alzheimer's Association. Alzheimer's Disease facts and figures. Alzheimers Dement 2009 May; 5(3):234–70.

Alzheimer's Association. Alzheimer's Disease facts and figures. Alzheimers Dement 2010 March; 6(2):158–94.

Alzheimer's Association: Recommendations to Update Diagnostic Criteria, accessible at http://www.alz.org/research/diagnostic%5Fcriteria/.

Alzheimer's Association and National Alliance for Caregiving. *FamiliesCare: Alzheimer's Caregiving in the United States, 2004*, accessible at www.alz.org.

American Heart Association: About Cholesterol, accessible at http://www.americanheart.org/presenter.jhtml?identifier=3046105.

American Psychiatric Association. Diagnostic and Statistical Manual of Mental Disorders (IV-TR). 4th edition-text revised. Washington, D.C., 2000.

Arvanitakis Z, Wilson RS, Bienias JL, Evans DA, Bennett DA. Diabetes mellitus and risk of Alzheimer disease and decline in cognitive function. Arch Neurol 2004 May; 61(5):661–66.

Bachurin S, Bukatina E, Lermontova N, et al. Antihistamine agent Dimebon as a novel nueroprotector and a cognition enhancer. Ann NY Acad Sci 2001; 939:425–35.

Biessels GJ, Kappelle LJ. Increased risk of Alzheimer's disease in type II diabetes: Insulin resistance of the brain or insulin-induced amyloid pathology? BST 2005; 33:1041–44.

Birks J. Cholinesterase inhibitors for Alzheimer's disease. Cochrane Database Syst Rev 2006 Jan 25; 1:CD00593.

Birks J, Grimley Evans J. Ginkgo biloba for cognitive impairment and dementia. Cochrane Database Syst Rev 2009 Jan 21; 1:CD003120.

Boller F, Forbes MM. History of dementia and dementia in history: An overview. Journal of the Neurological Sciences 1998; 158:125–33.

Canon, Lou. "Actor, Governor, President, Icon." *Washington Post*, June 6, 2004, page A1.

Center for Disease Control: Traumatic Brain Injury, accessible at http://www.cdc.gov/ncipc/factsheets/tbi.htm.

Centers for Medicare and Medicaid Services, accessible at https://www.cms.gov/.

Cochrane JJ, et al. The mental health of informal caregivers in Ontario: An epidemiological survey. Am J Public Health 1997; 87:2002–7.

Corkin S. What's new with the amnesic patient H.M.? Nat Rev Neurosci 2002 Feb; 3(2):153–60.

Craig-Schapiro R, Fagan AM, Holtzman DM. Biomarkers of Alzheimer's disease. Neurobiology of Disease 2009; 35:128–40.

Crum RM, Anthony JC, Bassett SS, Folstein MF. Population-based norms for the Mini-Mental State Examination by age and educational level. JAMA 1993; 269:2386.

Devore EE, et al. Dietary intake of fish and omega-3 fatty acids in relation to long-term dementia risk. Am J Clin Nutri 2009 Jul; 90(1):170–76.

Doody RS, Gavrilova SI, Sano M, et al. Effect of dimebon on cognition, activities of daily living, behavior, and global function in patients with mild-to-moderate Alzheimer's disease: A randomized, double-blind, placebo-controlled study. Lancet 2008; 372(9634):207–15.

Exley C, Esiri MM. Severe cerebral congophilic angiopathy coincident with increased brain aluminium in a resident of Camelford, Cornwall, UL. J Neurol Neurosurg Psychiatry 2006; 77:977–79.

Féart C, Samieri C, Rondeau V, et al. Adherence to the Mediterranean diet, cognitive decline, and risk of dementia. JAMA 2009; 302(6):638–48.

Feldman HH, Doody RS, Kivipelto M, et al. Randomized controlled trial of atorvastatin in mild to moderate Alzheimer disease: LEADe Neurology 2010; 74:956–64.

Fillit H, Hess G, Hill J, Bonnet P, Toso C. IV immunoglobulin is associated with a reduced risk of Alzheimer's disease and related disorders. Neurology 2009; 73:180–85.

Fischer P, et al. Conversion from subtypes of mild cognitive impairment to Alzheimer dementia. Neurology 2007; 68:288–91.

Folstein MF, Folstein, SE, McHugh, PR. Mini-mental state: A practical method for grading the cognitive state of patients for the clinician. J Psychiatr Res 1975; 12:189.

Food and Drug Administration: Antipsychotics, Conventional and Atypical, accessible at http://www.fda.gov/Safety/MedWatch/SafetyInformation/SafetyAlertsforHuman MedicalProducts/ucm110212.htm.

Franklin Institute. Blood Vessels in the Human Heart, accessible at http://www.fi.edu/learn/heart/vessels/vessels.html.

Fratiglioni L, Paillard-Borg S, Winblad B. An active and socially integrated lifestyle in late life might protect against dementia. Lancet Neurol 2004 Jun; (6):343–53.

Frisardi V, et al. Aluminum in the diet and Alzheimer's disease: from current epidemiology to possible disease-modifying treatment. J Alzheimers Dis 2010 Apr; 20(1): 17–30.

Gatz M, et al. Role of genes and environments for explaining Alzheimer disease. Arch Gen Psychiatry 2006 Feb; 63(2):168–74.

Gazzaley AH, Weiland NG, McEwen BS, Morrison JH. Differential regulation of NMDAR1 mRNA and protein by estradiol in the rat hippocampus. J Neurosci 1996 Nov 1; 16(21):6830–38.

Gearing M, Mirra SS, Hedreen JC, Sumi SM, Hansen LA, Heyman A. The Consortium to Establish a Registry for Alzheimer's Disease (CERAD). Part X. Neuropathology confirmation of the clinical diagnosis of Alzheimer's disease. Neurology 1995 Mar; 45(3 Pt 1):461–66.

Gispen WH, Biessels GJ. Cognition and synaptic plasticity in diabetes mellitus. Trends Neurosci 2000; 23:542–49.

Haag MD, Hofman A, Koudstaal PJ, Stricker BH, Breteler MM. Statins are associated with a reduced risk of Alzheimer disease regardless of lipophilicity: The Rotterdam Study. J Neurol Neurosurg Psychiatry 2009; 80:13–17.

Herbert LE, et al. Alzheimer disease in the US population: prevalence estimates using the 2000 census. Arch Neurol 2003; 60:1119–22.

Hogervorst E, Yaffe K, Richards M, Huppert FA. Hormone replacement therapy to maintain cognitive function in women with dementia. Cochrane Database Syst Rev 2009 Jan 21; 1:CD003799.

Imbimbo BP. An update on the efficacy of non-steroidal anti-inflammatory drugs in Alzheimer's disease. Expert Opin Investig Drugs 2009 August; 18(8):1147–68.

Irie F, Fitzpatrick AL, Lopez OL, Kuller LH, Peila R, Newman AB, Launer LJ. Enhanced risk for Alzheimer's disease in person with type 2 diabetes and apoe4: The cardiovascular health study cognition study. Arch Neuol 2008 Jan; 65(1):89–93.

Isaac MG, Quinn R, Tabet N. Vitamin E for Alzheimer's disease and mild cognitive impairment. Cochrane Database Syst Rev 2008 Jul 16; 3:CD002854.

Kawas CH. Clinical practice. Early Alzheimer's disease. N Engl J Med 2003 Sep 11; 349(11):1056–63.

Knopman DS, Boeve BF, Peterson RC. Essentials of the proper diagnosis of mild cognitive impairment, dementia, and major subtypes of dementia. Mayo Clin Proc 2003 Oct; 78(10):1290–308.

Lancelot E, Beal MF. Glutamate toxicity in chronic neurodegenerative disease. Prog Brain Res 1998; 116:331.

Leverenz JB, Raskind MA. Early amyloid deposition in the medial temporal lobe of young Down syndrome patients: a regional quantitative analysis. Exp Neurol 1998; 150:296–304.

Lindvall O, Kokaia Z. Stem cells in human neurodegenerative disorders—time for clinical translation? J Clin Invest 2010; 120(1):29–40.

Lott IT, Head E. Alzheimer's disease and Down syndrome: Factors in pathogenesis. Neurobiology of Aging 2005; 26:383–89.

Luine VN. Estradiol increases choline acetyltransferase activity in specific basal forebrain nuclei and projection areas of female rats. Exp Neurol 1985 Aug; 89(2):484–90.

Maurer Konrad, et al. Auguste D and Alzheimer's disease. Lancet 1997; 349: 1546–49.

McCurry SM, et al. Nighttime insomnia treatment and education for Alzheimer's disease: A randomized, controlled trial. J Am Geriatr Soc 2005 May; 53(5):793–802.

McKhann G, Drachman D, Folstein M, Katzman R, Price D, Stadlan EM. Clinical diagnosis of Alzheimer's disease: report of the NINCDS-ADRDA Work Group under the auspices of Department of Health and Human Services Task Force on Alzheimer's Disease. Neurology 1984 Jul; 34(7):939–44.

McShane R, et al. Memantine for dementia. Cochrane Database Syst Rev 2006 Apr 19; 2:CD003154.

Medivation. Pfizer and Medivation Announce Results from Two Phase 3 Studies in Dimebon (Latrepirdine*) Alzheimer's Disease Clinical Development Program, 2010, accessible at http://investors.medivation.com/releasedetail.cfm?ReleaseID=448818.

National Institute on Aging, accessible at http://www.nia.nih.gov/Alzheimers/Publica tions/Unraveling/Part1/.

Ngandu T, von Strauss E, Helkala EL, Winblad B, Nissinen A, Tuomilehto J, Soininen H, Kivipelto M. Education and dementia: What lies behind the association? Neurology 2007 Oct 2; 69(14):1442–50.

Nicola Lautenschlager, et al. Effect of physical activity on cognitive function in older adults at risk for Alzheimer's disease. JAMA 2008; 300:1027.

Phung TK, Andersen BB, Hogh P, Kessing LV, Mortensen PB, Waldemar G. Validity of dementia diagnoses in the Danish hospital registers. Dement Geriatr Cogn Disord 2007; 24(3):220–28. Epub 2007 Aug 10.

Qaseem A, et al. Current pharmacologic treatment of dementia: A clinical practice guideline from the American College of Physicians and the American Academy of Family Physicians. Ann Intern Med 2008 Mar 4; 148(5):370–78.

Querfurth HW, LaFerla FM. Alzheimer's disease. N Engl J Med 2010; 362:329–44.

Rafii MS, Aisen PS. Recent developments in Alzheimer's disease therapeutics. BMC Medicine 2009; 7:7.

Rapp SR, et al. Effect of estrogen plus progestin on global cognitive function in postmenopausal women: the Women's Health Initiative Memory Study: a randomized controlled trial. JAMA 2003 May 28; 289(20):2663–72.

Reisberg B, Doody R, Stöffler A, Schmitt F, Ferris S, Möbius HJ, Memantine Study Group. Memantine in moderate-to-severe Alzheimer's disease. N Engl J Med 2003 Apr 3; 348(14):1333–41.

Reitz C, Tang MX, Luchsinger J, Mayeux R. Relation of plasma lipids to Alzheimer's disease and vascular dementia. Arch Neurol 2004 May; 61(5):705–14.

Roberts GW, Gentleman SM, Lynch A, Murray L, Landon M, Graham DI. Beta-amyloid protein deposition in the brain after severe head injury: implications for the pathogenesis of Alzheimer's disease. J Neurol Neurosurg, Psychiatry 1994 57:419–25.

Rowe MA, et al. Persons with dementia who become lost in the community: A case study, current research, and recommendations. Mayo Clin Proc 2004 Nov; 79(11): 1417–22.

Rudelli R, Strom JO, Welch PT, Ambler MW. Post-traumatic premature Alzheimer's disease. Arch Neuro 1982 Sep; 39(9):570–75.

Salloway S, Sperling R, MD, Gilman S, Fox NC, Blennow K, Raskind M, Sabbagh M, Honig LS, Doody R, van Dyck CH, Mulnard R, Barakos J, Gregg KM, Liu E, Lieberburg I, Schenk D, Black R, Grundman M. For the Bapineuzumab 201 clinical trial investigators. A phase 2 multiple ascending dose trial of bapineuzumab in mild to moderate Alzheimer's disease. Neurology 2009; 73:2061–70.

Sampson EL, et al. Enteral tube feeding for older people with advanced dementia. Cochrane Database Syst Rev 2009 Apr 15; 2:CD007209.

Saunders AM, Strittmatter WJ, Schmechel D, et al. Association of apolipoprotein E allele epsilon 4 with late-onset familial and sporadic Alzheimer's disease. Neurology 1993; 43:1467–72.

Scarmeas N, et al. Mediterranean diet and mild cognitive impairment. Arch Neurol 2009 Feb; 66(2):216–25.

Scarmeas N, Luchsinger JA, Schupf N, et al. Physical activity, diet, and risk of Alzheimer disease. JAMA 2009; 302(6):627–37.

Schneider JA. High blood pressure and microinfarcts: A link between vascular risk factors, dementia, and clinical Alzheimer's disease. J Am Geriatr Soc 2009 Nov; 57(11): 2146–47.

Schneider LS, et al. Risk of death with atypical antipsychotic drug treatment for dementia: Meta-analysis of randomized placebo-controlled trials. JAMA 2005 Oct 19; 294(15):1934–43.

Schulz R, Beach SR, Lind B, Martire LM, Zdaniuk B, Hirsch C, Jackson S, Burton L . Involvement in caregiving and adjustment to death of a spouse: Findings from the caregiver health effects study. JAMA, 2001 June 27; 285(24):3123–9.

Sink KM, et al. Pharmacological treatment of neuropsychiatric symptoms of dementia: A review of the evidence. JAMA 2005 Feb 2; 293(5): 596–608.

Solomon A, Kareholt I, Ngandu T, Winblad B, Nissinen A, Tuomilehto J, Soininen H, Kiyipelto M. Serum cholesterol changes after midlife and late-life cognition: Twenty-one-year follow-up study. Neurology 2007 Mar 6; 68(10):751–56.

Stephen R. Rapp, et al. Effect of estrogen plus progestin on global cognitive function in postmenopausal women: the Women's Health Initiative Memory Study: A randomized controlled trial. JAMA 2003; 289:2663.

Stern Y, Gurland B, Taternichi TK, Tang MX, Wilder D, Mayeux R. Influence of education and occupation on the incidence of Alzheimer's disease. JAMA 1994 Apr 6; 271(13):1004–10.

Tanzi RE. A genetic dichotomy model for the inheritance of Alzheimer's disease and common age-related disorders. J Clin Invest 1999; 104:1175–79.

Tariot PN, Farlow MR, Grossberg GT, Graham SM, McDonald S, Gergel I. Memantine treatment in patients with moderate to severe Alzheimer's disease already receiving donepezil: A randomized controlled trial. JAMA 2004; 291:317–24.

Thomas, Evan. "Questions of Aged and Competence." *Time*, October 22, 1984, page 3.

U.S. Census Bureau. "U.S. Interim Projections by Age, Sex, Race, and Hispanic Origin: 2000–2050" in Population Projections, accessible at: http://www.census.gov/population/www/projections/usinterimproj/.

Van Den Heuvel C, Thornton E, Vink R. Traumatic brain injury and Alzheimer's disease: A review. Progress in Brain Research 2007; 161:303–16.

Watkins PB, et al. Hepatotoxic effects of tacrine administration in patients with Alzheimer's disease. JAMA 1994 Apr 6; 271(13):992–98.

Wierenga CE, Bondi MW. Use of functional magnetic resonance imaging in the early identification of Alzheimer's disease. Neuropsychol Rev 2007; 17:127–43.

Wilson RS, Li Y, Aggarwal NT, Barnes LL, McCann JJ, Gilley DW, Evans DA. Education and the course of cognitive decline in Alzheimer disease. Neurology 2004 Oct 12; 63(7):1198–202.

World Health Organization, Alzheimer's Disease: The Brain Killer, accessible at http://www.searo.who.int/EN/Section1174/Section1199/Section1567/Section1823_8066.htm.

Yesavage JA, Brink TL, Rose TL, Lum O, Huang V, Adey MB, Leirer VO: Development and validation of a geriatric depression screening scale: A preliminary report. Journal of Psychiatric Research 1983; 17:37–49.

# Index

Abstract thinking, impaired, 36–37
Acetylcholine, 61–62
Activities of Daily Living (ADL), 46
Adult day care, 96, 99–100
Age, as risk factor, 4–5, 18
Agitation and aggression, 69–73
Agnosia, 41–42, 47
Alcoholic dementia, 25
Alcohol use, 25, 46
Aluminum exposure, 15–16
Alzheimer, Alois, 1–2, 3, 10, 11
Alzheimer's disease: cost of, 5–6; defined, 2; described, 1–4; geographic differences in reported cases, 4; learning about, 96–97; number of people with, 4. *See also specific topics*
American Psychiatric Association, 41
Amygdala, 8
Amyloid plaques, 10–11, 12

Amyloid precursor proteins (APP), 10, 17
Anemia, 53
Antidepressants, 67
Antipsychotic drugs, 72–73
Aphasia, 41
Apolipoprotein E (ApoE), 17, 53
APP (amyloid precursor proteins), 10, 17
Apraxia, 41, 47
Aricept (donepezil), 61–63
Aspiration, 87
Assisted living, 101
Atypical antipsychotics, 73
Auditory hallucinations, 71
Auguste D. (patient), 1–2, 3, 10, 11
Axons, 7, 61

Bapineuzumab, 106
Behavioral symptom management, 66–76; agitation and aggression,

69–73; depression, 66–67; sleep, 67–69; wandering, 74–76

Behavior changes, 35, 84–85

Beta-amyloids, 10–11, 15, 17

Biomarkers, 104

Blood count, 53

Blood pressure, high, 20–21, 22, 48

Blood tests, 52–55

Blood vessels, 7, 19–20

Boxers, 18, 19

Brain: changes in, 10–12; structure and functions, 6–10

Brain imaging, 55–57, 104–5

Caregiver burden, 91, 93–94

Caregivers: coping tips, 93–96; mild disease and, 82–83; moderate disease and, 85; resources and support for, 78, 96–102; severe disease and, 87, 88; sleep disturbances and, 67, 68–69; unpaid, 5–6; wandering and, 74–75

Case managers, 98

CAT (computed tomography) scans, 56, 57

Causes. *See* Risk factors

Cerebrum, 7, 8

Cholesterol, high, 21, 22

Cholesterol-lowering medications, 109

Cholinesterase inhibitors, 61–63

Chromosome 21, 17

Cognex (tacrine), 61

Cognitive abilities, decline in, 41–42, 43, 47

Cognitive reserve, 23–24

Communication difficulties, 30–31

Computed tomography (CT) scans, 56, 57

Coordination, loss of, 33

Cost of Alzheimer's disease, 5–6

Counting, difficulty with, 37

Course and complications, 79–88; early disease, 80; mild disease, 80–83; moderate disease, 83–86; overview, 3–4, 12, 79–80; severe disease, 86–88

Cranial nerve exam, 49

Cross, Mrs. (patient), 15

CT (computed tomography) scans, 56, 57

D., Auguste (patient), 1–2, 3, 10, 11

Day care, adult, 96, 99–100

Delirium, 51–52

Delusions, 70, 71, 72

Dementia: defined, 2; diagnosis, 42, 50–51; in history, 79. *See also* Alzheimer's disease

Dementia pugilistica, 18–19

Dendrites, 7

Depression, 52, 66–67

Diabetes, 22–23

Diagnosis, 39–58; brain imaging, 55–57, 104–5; of dementia, 42, 50–51; diagnostic criteria, 41–43; history taking, 43–47; importance of, 60; laboratory tests, 52–55; neuropsychological testing, 57–58; overview, 39–41; physical exam, 47–52; research on, 103–5

*Diagnostic and Statistical Manual of Mental Disorders, Fourth Edition* (DSM-IV), 41, 43

Diagnostic criteria, 41–43

Diet, 25, 76–77, 109

Dimebon, 105–6

Disorientation, 31–32, 81–82

Donepezil (Aricept), 61–63

Down syndrome, 17

Driving abilities, 36, 85–86

Drugs. *See* Medications, in history taking; Pharmacologic management

Early disease, 80

Early-onset familial Alzheimer's disease, 17

Education, as risk factor, 23–24

Electrolytes, 53–54

Emotional impact on family, 92
Estrogen replacement, 25, 108
Executive function, 42
Exelon (rivastigmine), 61–63
Extrapyramidal symptoms, 73

Familial/genetic risk factors, 16–17, 46
Family, impact on, 90–93; emotional impact, 92; financial impact, 91–92; health impact, 90–91; physical impact, 93
Family history, 46
Feeding tubes, 76–77
Financial impact on family, 91–92
First generation antipsychotics, 73
Fish oil, 108–9
Forgetfulness, 27, 28–29, 80
Frontal lobe, 8
Frontotemporal dementia, 57
Functional history, 46–47
Functional MRI, 104–5

Gait assessment, 49–50
Gait disturbance, 77–78, 85, 86
Galantamine (Razadyne), 61–63
Gamma-secretase, 106
Genetic/familial risk factors, 16–17, 46
Geographic differences in reported cases, 4
Geriatric case managers, 98
Geriatric Depression Scale (GDS), 52
Geriatric social workers, 98
Ginkgo biloba, 108
Glial cells, 7
Glutamate, 63–64

Hallucinations, 70–71, 72
Head injury, 18–19
Health impact on family, 90–91
Hearing hallucinations, 71
Heart rate, 48
Help: accepting, 98–99; in-home, 100–101

Hippocampus, 8–10, 12
History taking, 43–47; family history, 46; functional history, 46–47; history of present illness, 43–44; medications, 44–45; past medical history, 44; social history, 45–46
H.M. (patient), 9–10
Homocysteine, 25
Hormone replacement therapy, 25, 108
Hypercholesterolemia, 21, 22
Hyperlipidemia, 21, 22
Hypertension, 20–21, 22, 48
Hypothalamus, 10
Hypothyroidism, 54

IADL (Instrumental Activities of Daily Living), 46–47
Impulse control, loss of, 84–85
Incontinence, 87
Infections, 88
Initiative, loss of, 35
Insight, lack of, 82
Instrumental Activities of Daily Living (IADL), 46–47
Intravenous immunoglobulin (IVIG), 106

Judgment, poor, 35–36

Kidney function tests, 53

Laboratory tests, 52–55
Language problems, 30–31, 82, 83–84, 86–87
Late-onset Alzheimer's disease, 17
Lifestyle risk factors, 23–25
Limbic system, 8–10
Liver function tests, 54
Long-term memory, 29–30

M., H. (patient), 9–10
Magnetic resonance imaging (MRI) scans, 56, 57, 104–5

Medical history, past, 44
Medications, in history taking, 44–45.
    *See also* Pharmacologic management
Memantine (Namenda), 63–65
Memory loss: as diagnostic criterion, 41,
    42–43; as sign, 28–30, 80–81, 83
Mental activities/engagement, 23–25,
    109
Mental status exam, 50–51
Metabolic syndrome, 22
Mild cognitive impairment, 42
Mild disease, 80–83
Mini-Mental State Exam (MMSE),
    50–51, 57, 64
Moderate disease, 83–86
Mood changes, 34–35
Motor exam, 49
MRI (magnetic resonance imaging) scans,
    56, 57, 104–5

Namenda (memantine), 63–65
Napping, 68
National Institute of Neurological and
    Communicative Disorders and Stroke
    and the Alzheimer's Disease and
    Related Disorders Association
    (NINCDS-ADRDA), 41, 43
Nerve cells, 6–7, 61
Neurofibrillary tangles, 11, 12
Neuroimaging, 55–57, 104–5
Neurologic exam, 49–51
Neurons, 6–7, 61
Neuropsychological testing, 57–58
Neurotransmitters, 7, 61
N-methyl-D-aspartate (NMDA) recep-
    tors, 63–64
Nonsteroidal anti-inflammatory drugs
    (NSAIDs), 108
Nursing homes, 101–2
Nursing services, in-home, 100
Nutrition, 25, 76–77, 109

Objects, misplaced, 29
Occipital lobe, 8
Occupational therapists, 100–101
Omega-3 fatty acids, 108–9

Parietal lobe, 8
Personality changes, 33–34, 82
PET (positron emission tomography)
    scans, 105
Pharmacologic management, 61–65;
    cholinesterase inhibitors, 61–63;
    memantine, 63–65; other medications,
    65; research on, 105–7
Physical exam, 47–52; delirium, 51–52;
    depression, 52; described, 48–49;
    mental status exam, 50–51; neurologic
    exam, 49–51; vital signs, 47–48
Physical exercise/activity, 23, 24–25, 109
Physical impact on family, 93
Physical therapists, 100
Planning: by caregivers for future, 97–98;
    patient difficulty with, 37
Positron emission tomography (PET)
    scans, 105
Prevention, research on, 107–9
Punch drunk syndrome, 18–19

Razadyne (galantamine), 61–63
Reagan, Ronald, 27, 30
Research, 103–9; diagnostic tools,
    103–5; overview, 103; prevention of
    Alzheimer's disease, 107–9; treatment
    of Alzheimer's disease, 105–7
Resources and support for caregivers, 78,
    96–102
Respite care, 96
Rest and health, finding time for, 94–95
Risk factors, 15–26; age, 4–5, 18; diabe-
    tes, 22–23; familial/genetic, 16–17;
    head injury, 18–19; hyperlipidemia, 21,
    22; hypertension, 20–21, 22; lifestyle,

23–25; other, 25–26; overview, 15–16; vascular, 19–23
Rivastigmine (Exelon), 61–63
Robinson, Sugar Ray, 18
Routines, 69, 71–72

Second generation antipsychotics, 73
Semagacestat, 106
Sensory exam, 49
Severe disease, 86–88
Short-term memory, 29, 30
Side effects of medications, 44–45
Signs, 27–37; abstract thinking, impaired, 36–37; disorientation, 31–32, 81–82; judgment, poor, 35–36; language problems, 30–31, 82, 83–84, 86–87; memory loss, 28–30, 80–81, 83; mood and behavior changes, 34–35, 84–85; overview, 27; personality changes, 33–34, 82; tasks, difficulty with familiar, 32–33, 81, 83–84
Skilled nursing, 101–2
Skin ulcers, 87–88
Sleep disturbances, 67–69
Sleeping medications, 69
Smoking, 25, 46
Social activities/engagement, 23, 24–25, 109
Social history, 45–46
Social workers, 98
Statins, 109
Stroke, 57
Sun-downing, 70, 84
Support groups, 95
Swallowing difficulties, 76

Synapse, 7
Syphilis, 55

Tacrine (Cognex), 61
Tasks, difficulty with familiar, 32–33, 81, 83–84
Tau proteins, 11, 104, 107
Temporal lobe, 8
Thalamus, 10
Therapists, 95
Thyroid function tests, 54
Thyroid gland, underactive, 54
Treatment, 59–78; behavioral symptom management, 66–76; caregivers support, 78; gait disturbance, 77–78; nutrition, 76–77; overview, 59–60; pharmacologic management, 61–65; research on, 105–7
Trisomy 21, 17
Twin studies, 16–17
Typical antipsychotics, 73

"Up and Go Test," 49–50

Vascular risk factors, 19–23; diabetes, 22–23; hyperlipidemia, 21, 22; hypertension, 20–21, 22, 48
Visual hallucinations, 71
Vital signs, 47–48
Vitamin B12, 54–55
Vitamin E, 107–8

Wandering, 74–76, 85
Weight loss, unintentional, 48, 76–77
Word-finding problems, 30, 31

## About the Authors

**LINDA C. LU,** MD, is an Associate Physician at Brigham and Women's Hospital and an Instructor in Medicine at Harvard Medical School. Dr. Lu received her medical degree from New York Medical College and completed her residency in internal medicine at the UCLA-VA. She went on to complete a Clinical Fellowship in Geriatric Medicine at Harvard Medical School. Areas of interest include caring for the oldest and frailest in the community.

**JUERGEN H. BLUDAU,** MD, received his medical degree from the Royal College of Surgeons in Ireland and completed his postgraduate studies in the USA. He is a board-certified, Harvard fellowship-trained geriatrician, and currently the Acting Clinical Chief and Director of the clinical geriatric services at the Brigham and Women's Hospital, Division of Aging. Dr. Bludau is an Instructor in Medicine at Harvard Medical School, and a member of the Scientific Advisory Board of the Gerontological Economic Research Organization in Kreuzlingen, Switzerland.

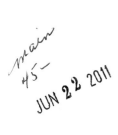